Health, Trade and Human Rights

D1147693

Théodore H MacDonald

*Professor (emeritus), formerly Director of Postgraduate Studies in
Health, Brunel University; Associate of the Institute of Human
Rights and Social Justice, Metropolitan University of London;
Fellow, Royal Society of Medicine*

Forewords by

Mogobe Ramose

and

Desmond M Tutu

Radcliffe Publishing
Oxford • Seattle

Radcliffe Publishing Ltd
18 Marcham Road
Abingdon
Oxon OX14 1AA
United Kingdom

www.radcliffe-oxford.com
Electronic catalogue and worldwide online ordering facility.

British Library Cataloguing in Publication data

A catalogue record for this book is available from the British Library.

ISBN-10 1 84619 050 9
ISBN-13 978 1 84619 050 6

Typeset by Advance Typesetting Ltd, Oxford
Printed and bound by TJ International Ltd, Padstow, Cornwall

Contents

Foreword

Welcome to the world of Théodore MacDonald. It is the world of a man with vast experience in health matters around the globe. In his case, experience, critically examined, is the best teacher. His experience is deeply involved with the mistress of science in a way that speaks to the person in the street, the activist, the theoretician and the politician. This combination of experience with scientific rigour is presented in accessible everyday language. It is seductive, inviting the curiosity of the reader to last until the very end of the book.

It is also the world of a man who discerns the intricate connections between health matters and the politics of wealth. MacDonald goes beyond discernment by having the courage to criticise the basis, the method and the extent to which the politics of wealth continues to undermine and violate the right of the poor to good health. Thus neither the title of this book nor the sequence of its wording is accidental. Placing *health* as the first word in the title speaks directly to the famous saying that preserving the good health of the people is the supreme law of the state. Unsurprisingly MacDonald then demonstrates that Cuba is much more obedient to this saying than the United States of America.

MacDonald demonstrates that the nature and practice of trade under the regimes of the International Monetary Fund, the World Bank and the World Trade Organization are a crime against the law of the preservation of the good health of the people, in particular the poor. The remedy to this is the replacement of the illusion of free trade with the reality of fair trade. His argument necessitates that *trade* should be the second word of the title.

Good health preserves human life. It recognises and respects the dignity of the person as a human being. It is the admission that the right to life is primary and paramount. MacDonald demonstrates that the dogma of free trade in fact violates this right in respect of the poor. The book is dedicated to Ken Saro Wiwa who, in part, demanded fair trade for his people. His demand reaffirms the necessity to recognise, respect and protect the right to life of all human beings by dismantling the edifice of structural poverty. The human rights discourse will remain empty and problematical for as long as it sidesteps this re-affirmation. MacDonald's argument here echoes at the right time the famous declaration of former American President John F Kennedy: 'if a free society cannot save the many who are poor, it cannot save the few who are rich'. So *human rights* follows logically as the third term in the title of this book. Obviously, this does not mean, for critical MacDonald, that human rights is the third in an imaginary order of priority.

MacDonald's courage to criticise is tempered with his deep and admirable sense of fairness. He is sharply and correctly critical of America's apparent resolution to weaken the United Nations and subordinate it to the pursuit of her national interest. At the same time he is careful to advise that there are Americans who are critical of the policies and actions of their leaders. It is such Americans who deserve support and solidarity with the rest of humankind, demanding action in the sphere of social justice instead of obsequious reverence for grand declarations of policy.

The whole book is a discourse on ethics, urging humankind to take seriously our responsibility towards ourselves and those yet to be born. The essence of this responsibility is that we should enjoy planet earth as much as we can before we depart from it – provided we make sure we leave it as good as we found it and leave enough in it for those yet to be born. Neglecting this responsibility in our interdependent and complex world means 'an early end to our existence'. This is not far-fetched doomsday pessimism if we consider the reality of the ever-present military threat of nuclear homicide.

Convinced of our ethical responsibility, MacDonald proposes some solutions to make our planet a true home of justice for all humankind. Thus he questions the sustainability of the profit motive in capitalism. Unlike George Soros, MacDonald argues for an alternative to capitalism. Like the Group of Lisbon, he decries the concept of 'competition' currently understood in capitalist economics. He proposes co-operation instead. Money is not always the root of evil. It is the purpose for which it is used that can become evil. MacDonald argues for a new concept of wealth based on the 'social good' capable of protecting and promoting the human dignity of every member of society. This cannot come about without the recovery of the lost sense of community, especially in the West. He therefore urges the West and the rest of humankind to take the philosophy and practice of *ubuntu* seriously in the endeavour to recover the meaning of community.

MacDonald argues further that the changes required do not need resort to war. This is a particularly pertinent point since the military reality of our time demands that we recognise the irrationality of war, even if it is non-nuclear war. Thus MacDonald makes a strong plea for a 'revolutionary' change of mindset oriented towards the practical realisation of social justice. MacDonald's message is clear and unambiguous: war is no longer the father of all things. Instead, justice is the mother of all peace.

Mogobe Ramose
Chair, Department of Philosophy
University of South Africa
Tshwane
South Africa
December 2005

Foreword

The present book is a natural sequel to the author's *Third World Health: Hostage to First World Wealth*, and what I said in the Foreword to that book applies with equal force to this one. My country was, until the end of apartheid rule, regarded by many as a 'third-world' nation because of the way in which the great majority of its citizens were compelled to live. Of course, it was not a third-world nation for the white minority, most of whom enjoyed enviable health and educational facilities and a high economic standard of life. South Africa is still, in many respects, a third-world nation, ravaged by HIV/AIDS (human immunodeficiency virus/acquired immune deficiency syndrome), and we are progressing only slowly in overcoming many of the deficits of our once divided society. I therefore identify with many of the issues raised in this book. The author's thorough analysis of the HIV/AIDS pandemic in Africa and elsewhere is not only statistically sound but intimately reflects his concern with the need for international equity.

As we draw to the end of the year 2005, South Africa, along with many other parts of the world, still faces enormous problems due to inequity, both within and between nations. I call to mind the words of the prophet Isaiah in Chapter 35, when he speaks of the coming of God to his people – 'the desert shall rejoice and bloom as the rose (v.i) say to those that are of fearful heart: "Be strong, fear not ... your God will save you" (v.iv) and the people obtain joy and gladness, and sorrow and sighing shall die away' (v.x). We in South Africa have won freedom from apartheid. Are we now to face ruin and desertification, disease and terror? The answer to that question, as Théodore makes clear in this book, is very much up to us. We live in a world in which a large proportion of the world's people are condemned to live on less than one US dollar a day, where HIV/AIDS and other preventable diseases create millions of orphans and in which the already economically deprived nations are driven further into privation by unfair trading practices imposed in the interests of the already rich and powerful. But, as this book makes clear, we can make the world a place in which the desert shall bloom, justice reign and the people know joy and gladness.

As the author clearly illustrates, a basic problem underlying such inequalities in health between the first and the third world centres on globalised first-world control of trade. The poor nations are being forced to accede to the dictates of 'free trade' rather than 'fair trade', thus exposing their populations to even greater impoverishment and ill health. MacDonald shows how even the World Health Organization (WHO) – which at its outset promoted health as a 'basic human right' – has been forced to acquiesce to World Trade Organization (WTO) pressure to let health become subject to multilateral instruments such as the General Agreement on Trade in Services. Thus, increasingly, people's health is no longer a basic human right but a trade-related commodity.

Théodore MacDonald writes with passion, as well as with sense. Much of what he has to say is drawn from his own experience working as a medical doctor and a mathematician in a broad range of the world's poorest nations. But overarching that is a powerful insight into social and economic issues, along with well-honed skills as a communicator. His thorough knowledge of history and politics has enabled him to contextualise what he has witnessed and laboured to remedy. His writing style is astonishingly accessible, informing and inspiring the lay reader as much as the professional. The analyses underpinning both his exposition and his arguments are penetratingly accurate and embrace a wide readership. It is regrettable but true that many books which address the issues herein from a position committed to equity are under-powered with respect to evidence and analytical rigour. Such certainly does not characterise the present volume.

The author deals in an admirably balanced style with vexatious issues which, in less experienced hands, could easily lead to shrill political rhetoric and narrow sectarian argument. But MacDonald clearly feels that the issues are far too important for ideological point-scoring. To him, the crucial thing is to equip the reader, lay or professional, not only with the facts but also with an insight into how they came about. Readers are often made aware of some particularly outrageous violation of human rights with respect to international trade – and the enormous health and social deficits which ensue – but this book allows us to see beyond these particulars to the consequences of sitting back and doing nothing. MacDonald persuades us of our power to influence local events, to develop an informed community stance on environmental issues, etc.

In discussing solutions, the author strongly makes the point that it is too easy to allow one's commitment to global justice to be siphoned off into something completely negative, like anti-Americanism. As he points out, the USA is the most powerful nation on earth and has a history of sustained commitment to the values of democracy, accountability and justice. MacDonald argues that we need to delve behind the actions of some of its large corporations, the globalisation of finance under terms favourable to corporate greed and exploitation. As a nation, the USA has contributed, and continues to do so, massively to human culture and civilisation. It is a repository of so many positive values, achievements and of so much creativity. The problem, argues the author, is not the dominance of one particular country in global economic affairs, but is our failure so far to truly transcend national interests in response to global needs. It was for that very purpose that the United Nations was established. But that organisation is often powerless under present rules governing it. It cannot intervene effectively without real transnational authority in areas such as health, education and other human rights. MacDonald suggests ways around this problem in which global mediation of such basic human rights as health can be based on 'geographic zones' rather than specific nations, with the emphasis on free trade within zones.

I am pleased to recommend this splendid book enthusiastically.

Desmond M Tutu
Archbishop Emeritus
Capetown
South Africa
December 2005

Preface

Trade between nations has always been intimately associated, both positively and negatively, with health. The positive aspects relate to widening the exchange of ideas and customs regarding health, the negative aspects with the introduction of diseases to which the native population has not developed immunity and/or the spread of lethal diseases such as bubonic plague or the ever-evolving virulent strains of influenza. It is also a truism that trade and imperialism are related because imperial powers have routinely organised trade with their colonies to the benefit of the former and the detriment of the latter. Therefore, the title of this book – *Health, Trade and Human Rights* – is rather self-explanatory. Throughout history empires have risen and fallen, and various peoples of the world have had their time at being colonies or imperial powers.

But the situation which prevails today is different in two crucial aspects.

- We now know the whole world. There are no unknown populations to exploit. For the first time, the most powerful hegemony the world has ever known is global. There is only one superpower – the USA at present – and just about all the other countries are either its uneasy first world satellites or belong to the third world. The control of global capitalism is increasingly widening the wealth gap (and, hence, the health and human rights gap) between the first world and the third. There is no natural cyclical process that is likely to reverse the steady trend to the benefit of an already advantaged first world over the steadily more disadvantaged third world. For the first time, finance is now globally mediated under neo-liberal (free trade, no localised protectionisms, etc.) orthodoxies. Thus, even if the present leading nation (the USA) should eventually give way to another, this will make no material difference to the issue of inbuilt inequities.
- The second major difference is rather more gothic. Never before in world history has there been a built-in timer mechanism on the growth of power. That 'timer' is none other than the environment, which is telling us with increasing urgency that we simply cannot continue as we have been. Environmental degradation and its consequences are rarely confined by national boundaries. Our

prodigious use of hydrocarbon fuels, for instance, to say nothing of the damage done to the environment in our relentless search for them, has brought us face to face, on the one hand, with global warming and its baleful effects, and, on the other, with an awareness of the finitude of the supply of such fuels.

For the first time we are actually forced, not by idealism, nor by religious faith, but by sheer political expediency, to realise that we inhabit a rather small planet and that we have to work together, as the human race, to preserve it and ourselves. This cannot possibly come about with one dominant power and one financial orthodoxy (neoliberalism) controlling trade and hence sustaining vast and increasing inequalities in health and other human rights between the first- and the third-world nations.

Events such as Bob Geldof's 'Live 8' give many people the impression that the third world is intrinsically poor. But this is not necessarily true. There are many valuable marketable resources in the third world, but the first world makes the global trading rules, effectively preventing the third world from exploiting its resources to the advantage of its own people. Remember Ken Saro Wiwa. Ken Saro Wiwa was murdered in 1995 for insisting that Nigeria was not poor. It only needed the freedom to exploit its own oil (and other national resources). His 'Movement for the Survival of the Ogoni People' demanded that Shell compensate for the US $30 billion of oil it pumped out of the country between 1955 and 1995. Consider this, Ken Saro Wiwa was executed by the Nigerian government – not by Shell. Yet Nigeria (the most modern and one of the largest and wealthiest of African countries) has about 67% of its people living (well, dying, really) on less than US $1 (70 pence UK) a day, as of 2004. But how can trade between unequally strong nations be mediated fairly? This is the main problem. To start with, it cannot realistically be mediated on the basis of 'free trade' arrangements with the richer nations' banks making the rules!

In this book, I give a coherent account as to how the present global system came into being after World War II, the origins and functions of the main financial bodies controlling trade, such as the International Monetary Fund (IMF), the World Bank and the World Trade Organization (WTO) and their various control mechanisms, such as structural adjustment policies (SAP), General Agreement on Tariffs and Trade (GATT), General Agreement on Trade in Services (GATS), various free trade and bilateral trade agreements and so forth. As a medical man, I have worked in a variety of third-world countries and have been able to monitor how these mechanisms for mediating trade to the advantage of shareholders in the first world actually affect health and human rights in the third world.

The book begins with a chapter in which I indicate certain broad categories of problems which militate against global equity. The United Nations (UN) Charter specifically identifies global equity in human rights as one of its aims and most countries in the world have signed up to that. I then devote a chapter to explaining how international trade is at present mediated and financed. Chapter 3 concerns itself primarily with environmental limitations to our activities. The next two chapters concern themselves with global health issues – breast milk substitutes and the frightful scourge of HIV/AIDS.

But each of these chapters explores in detail how the third world is so grotesquely disadvantaged in both of these global phenomena. As a counter to Chapter 1, Chapter 6 addresses various solutions to problems raised in the first chapter and argues a counsel of 'pro-active optimism'.

The problems we face can certainly no longer by regarded as 'academic' or 'theoretical'. We cannot even regard them as being 'remote' in the sense that they all involve faraway countries and people with whom we have little necessary involvement. Indeed, the present widespread concern about environmental issues, as dealt with in Chapter 3, abundantly illustrates how these concerns compel us all to be involved with one another. The problem with neo-liberal economics in practice is that, as presently mediated, it necessarily creates unsustainable discrepancies between populations in different parts of the planet. Any rational solution to the global environmental crisis means that we need to globalise human rights if we are to avert catastrophe.

Théodore MacDonald
December 2005

Acknowledgements

The writing of this book has involved the willing co-operation of legions of field-workers, medical staff, patients, government officials and others from whom the author was able to seek access to information. To them all, whether explicitly acknowledged in the text or not, a debt of thanks is owed. Without their aid and insights, much of this work could not have been completed. For sterling help in the word processing of the manuscript and the preparation of the charts, I thank Dr Hannah Caller and David Howarth.

The editorial staff of Radcliffe Publishing not only provided every encouragement but have exercised their usual thoroughness in editing the manuscript. Any imperfections in the content of the book are the sole responsibility of the author.

As usual, my wife, Chris, and my son, Matthew, were immensely supportive throughout the hectic turmoil of authorship!

To the memory of Ken Saro Wiwa (1941–1995), scholar, author and human rights activist in defence of the people of Nigeria's Ogoni Delta region in their struggle against the depredations of their land by international oil interests, and who was hanged by the Nigerian authorities for treason, this book is dedicated. As he was about to be hanged, he said:

'I'll tell you this. I may be dead but my ideas will not die!'

May his martyrdom to justice in trade be an inspiration to the rest of us in the continuing struggle against the tyranny of capitalism.

Chapter 1

What are the problems?

The link with imperialism

Christian scriptures teach us that 'The poor ye always have with you' (Matthew 26: 11), but they do not go on to say that the gap between the rich and poor of the world has been increasing almost uninterruptedly in the two millennia since Jesus reputedly uttered those words. In the early nineteenth century the hope and expectation among many European thinkers was that – with the benefits of science – the gap might soon begin to close. But the very reverse has happened. In fact, since the Industrial Revolution (say, from the 1760s) the poverty gap between the first and the third worlds has accelerated exponentially. The huge advantages conferred on the first world by computer technology and automation processes through the twentieth century have reflected themselves in an even greater rate of wealth differential between the rich and the poor. As this book will show, these phenomena are well documented and are evident even over comparatively short time intervals. For example, the proportion of people with access to safe water and rudimentary sanitation in rural Africa dropped from 60% in 2000 to only 43% by 2002. Indeed, in Africa's poorest countries income per person has fallen by 25% over the last 25 years (Matthiason and Townsend, 2005).

Of course, virtually from the beginning of recorded history (and no doubt before), trade and health have been inextricably linked, although the links were rarely anticipated beforehand, were often not observed for years after they had started to occur and were infrequently understood when they were observed. At the purely local level, one can cite many well-known examples – arsenic poisoning among tea-tasters in the seventeenth century, mercury poisoning associated with the haberdashery trade as late as the nineteenth century (viz. the Mad Hatter in Lewis Carroll's *Alice's Adventures in Wonderland*, published in 1865) (Dodgson, 1983). Even further back in time, we note the ruinous impact on the health of people who dyed togas in squid ink for the élite of the Roman Empire. We do not lack for examples.

As trade became international, and ineluctably associated with the imperialistic ventures of the industrialised world nations over much of the rest of the world, the link between trade and health became even more obvious. This was because, by and large, colonised peoples were accorded far fewer human rights than their masters enjoyed. They were given less protection from work-related accidents, poorer food and less of it. Also, the movement of ships and people from one part of the world to another facilitated the spread of disease. We only have to think of the dire impact of bubonic plague (the 'Black Death') even as far back as the fifth century BC in Greece.

But today such potentially negative effects of global trade on health are so much greater because of the ease, speed and volume of international air travel. Pandemics such as human immunodeficiency virus or acquired immune deficiency syndrome (HIV/AIDS) now threaten us all, as do various virulent forms of influenza, to say nothing of resurgent tuberculosis. It is sobering to remind the reader that, until the 1960s, many of us thought that tuberculosis had been effectively eradicated from Europe and North America.

European imperialism in Africa, Asia and the Americas, mainly between the sixteenth and nineteenth centuries, tended to create a situation in which the great bulk of such health problems impinged on the natives of colonised territories while, with astute planning and foresight, the majority of the benefits of trade accrued to the European moneyed classes. The eclipse of the major European colonial adventures (say, after 1945) did not see a reduction in these inequities. Rather, they have greatly increased. First-world corporations and governments have developed much more efficient forms of imperialism, most of it now controlled from the USA rather than from Europe. Without being too flippant, a US-based trans-national corporation can effectively subvert the entire economy of a third-world country by sending an e-mail between two banks. There is no more need of a globe-encircling navy or vast standing armies in garrisons all over the globe.

The negative effect on human rights (such as health, access to water and food, education and so on) through the exploitation of the third world to facilitate trade has been enormous. Subsequent chapters will deal more specifically with the details. Trade, for instance, has never been disassociated with war, but wars have been pretty well constant since 1945. Many of these conflicts are remote from first-world consciousness (our media is thoughtfully selective in this regard) and routinely the bulk of casualties are now borne by the civilian population rather than by the military.

Whose WHO?

The World Health Organization (WHO) was established as a United Nations (UN) body in the closing days of World War II and as a pivotal part of the UN's broader remit to oversee a more stable and just international order, with world peace and human rights as its major objectives. Health was unambiguously recognised as a 'basic human right', as was education. Universal access to health was seen as fundamental to this objective. Through the 1950s, 1960s and 1970s, the WHO was widely perceived as the vanguard of this noble enterprise, in which medically trained personnel from a variety of nations co-operated in defining international health agendas and in elaborating impressively successful drives against scourges such as poliomyelitis and smallpox. Among the director-generals of the WHO in those forward-looking days were such eminent figures as Dr GH Brundtland, Dr H Nakajima and Dr H Mahler. The latter, Dr Halfdan Mahler, in particular, was the energetic proponent of the 'Health for All 2000 (HFA 2000)' campaign, which emphasised primary healthcare* for all by the year 2000. This campaign was announced at the 1977 meeting of the World Health Assembly at Alma Ata in the Crimea, not far from Scutari where Florence Nightingale achieved such fame (WHO, 1978).

The underlying principles of primary healthcare were agreed at that meeting as follows.

- Universal access to healthcare on the basis of need alone.
- Care with the emphasis on prevention of disease and on personal and community health promotion.
- Full co-operation between various social and medical agencies in mediating healthcare. This is referred to as 'inter-sectorality' and

---

*Primary healthcare (as opposed to secondary or tertiary healthcare) technically refers to levels of technological sophistication and the infrastructures required for delivery, but, in the context of the WHO policy involved, it simply meant having healthcare available at the local community level to ensure unimpeded access.

can include a wide range of input – sporting, cultural, educational and so forth.

- Cost effectiveness at the administrative level (usually government-financed) and presenting no financial barrier to patient access.

Thirty-eight objectives were optimistically set out under the title 'Health for All 2000'. The aims were not achieved by 2000, not through any lack of commitment on the part of Mahler and his predecessors, but because by the late 1980s the WHO had already conceded too much ground to globalised financial initiatives, which regarded the interests of international trade as transcending health for all. Indeed, soon after Mahler retired from the WHO, the argument that primary healthcare is so costly that financial bases for trade to pay for it had to have priority was gaining favour. By 1989 it was generally realised that the 'Health for All 2000' objectives were not going to be met in time. Some of these were deferred until 2015, whereas others simply disappeared.

Truly, until the mid 1980s, the WHO seemed to transcend politics and commerce in pursuit of its heroic objectives. It was focused on the widespread application – to as many of the world's people as possible – of primary healthcare. Its methods were based purely on health needs and the elaboration of efficient means of meeting them.

At that time, then, the answer to the question: 'Whose WHO?' would have been 'Everyone's', but things have changed. After Mahler, the post of Director-General of the WHO has been held by people who felt that the aims and strategies of the WHO should be focused less on the meticulous collection of medical statistics as a basis for meeting clinical needs and more on optimising the affected nations' capacity to align their infrastructures with the needs of globalised trade and finance.

The situation is worse than this for, as we shall see in Chapter 2, nations are not even free to organise their trading relations within or between small blocs of contiguous territories, but increasingly must follow the dictates of the World Trade Organization (WTO). Without going into detail at this point, the WTO appears to be the ultimate expression of democracy in that every member country has equal voting rights. But the devil is in the detail, for there is no limit to the number of lawyers and other informed representatives that a country may send abroad to meetings (both formal and informal) to promote their nation's case. The USA can (and does) send out hundreds of such representatives, compared to every one (or none) in the case of many third-world nations. Very small nations, like St Lucia fighting for a fair share of the banana trade, are clearly at a great disadvantage. In most WTO mediations between claims from the USA and some smaller third-world country, the odds are overwhelmingly stacked in favour of US interests.

But what does the WTO have to do with the WHO, or with health generally? As previously noted, the WHO has found itself gradually moving away from its early 1980s stance on the primacy of health as a basic human right to one of health being necessarily subject to adjustments to nations' infrastructures as required by the needs of international trade. In other words, health is becoming seen as commodity that can be bargained for. It is now very much a matter of relative values and of political decisions with the WTO, rather than the WHO, calling the shots.

This is so much the case that, in the WTO Council, the WHO is only represented by a non-voting 'observer'. Trade, especially globalised trade, more often than not determines a poorer nation's 'rights' to health. So, in 2006, if we are faced with the question 'Whose WHO?', the answer is no longer 'Everyone's' but that of 'The bankers and capitalist corporations of the first world.'

Health planning for international trade

In this context let us consider the rather unwieldy terms 'horizontalisation' and 'verticalisation'. The first refers to the situation in which a nation sets out to mediate healthcare as promulgated at Alma Ata – as a basic human right applicable to as many of its people as possible. For instance, routine immunisation programmes, widespread access to mother and child clinics, universal sex and health education programmes in schools, and free and compulsory school attendance are examples of horizontalisation. It is routine in first-world nations, but is rare in the third world. Cuba is an outstanding counter-example to this (*see* Chapter 6). The second refers to a situation in which a nation concentrates its access to healthcare to those areas of the country most crucial to its trade and money-generating activities.

There are various third-world countries which have attempted to organise horizontalisation but which have eventually been compelled by World Bank and/or International Monetary Fund (IMF) debt repayment conditions (as discussed in Chapter 2) to give it up. Sometimes verticalisation has led to rather bizarre results. Take the case of Zambia, for instance. In 1973 a number of WHO reports were written trying to account for why antimalaria programmes, to which until 1970 malaria had been responding well in that country, were suddenly failing. It was found that the main reason was that Zambia, in order to meet the conditions for a loan from the IMF, had instituted verticalisation and hence terminated malaria control in rural areas (WHO, 1973). One could cite many other health inequities which arise from prioritising the needs of globalised trade, and some of these will be discussed in subsequent chapters. But, before specifying further problems as they affect third-world health, let us consider one immense problem which really involves an effective mechanism by which the first world is being massively aided financially by the third: the first world has been systematically using the third world as a reservoir of professionally trained health staff for its hospitals.

The 'brain drain' from the third to the first world

Any reader who has recently been a hospital patient in a major first-world city, such as London or New York, will have been struck by the high proportion of doctors and nurses, and other medical staff, who have had their training abroad. This author found, as a patient in some of London's leading hospitals, that a command of Spanish and/or Tagalog was almost a requirement in order to communicate with the large number of staff from the Philippines. Swahili and one or two West African languages would also not have gone amiss. In short, the UK's National Health Service (NHS), which serves its people so well, simply could not run without the huge corps of brilliantly trained and committed health professionals from the third world and for whose years of training we have not paid a penny.

The sheer injustice of this large-scale milking of the resources of poor countries desperately in need of their own medical staff has finally led various professional bodies in the UK to address the issue. For instance, the NHS no longer routinely sends recruitment teams to third-world countries in search of staff, but this does not prevent private agencies from doing so. Also, working conditions and pay are so much better in the UK and other first-world contexts that a high proportion of such staff head for first-world nations soon after completing their training. This is the sort of trans-national problem which must be addressed as part of any programme to promote human rights and social justice globally.

At the International People's Health University (IPHU), held in Ecuador in July 2005, Professor David Sanders, Director of the School of Public Health at the University of the Southern Cape in South Africa, presented figures which showed that the Organization for Economic Cooperation and Development (OECD)* countries have a workforce of about three million professionals who trained in the third world. Over the next 10 years, the USA alone is estimated to need 10 million more nurses. In the UK, the need is for 10 000 more doctors and 20 000 more nurses just to meet present healthcare plans. The question must surely arise as to just who is aiding whom?

Between 1985 and 1995, 60% of Ghana's medical graduates emigrated, whereas from 1990 to 2000, Zimbabwe lost a total of 840 of its 1200 medical graduates. In the year 2001, over 2000 South African nurses went to work in the UK. In financial terms the US government calculated that it made a saving of of about US$ 20 000 from each skilled worker who had trained in a third-world country (Sanders, 2005).

The health–wealth relationship

Even though health is regarded by the UN Charter as a basic human right (rather than a mere commodity), it should come as no great surprise that – generally speaking – the higher a nation's Gross National Income** (GNI), the higher will be its measure of health. To illustrate how close this correspondence is, consider the World Development Chart 2004 in Figure 1.1.

The chart shows the relationship between a country's GNI and one of the most commonly used health indices, namely the number of

---

*The Organization for Economic Cooperation and Development (OECD) countries can loosely be said to embrace the first world. Its aims include the promotion of trade, economic growth and aid to the third world. Its membership includes Australia, Austria, Belgium, Canada, the Czech Republic, Denmark, Finland, France, Germany, Greece, Hungary, Luxembourg, Mexico, the Netherlands, New Zealand, Norway, Poland, Portugal, Spain, Sweden, Switzerland, Turkey, the UK and the USA.
**Gross National Income (GNI) is calculated from Gross National Product (GNP), which in turn is defined as the total adjusted market value (in US dollars) of all the goods and services produced as income by a nation over a given period of time.

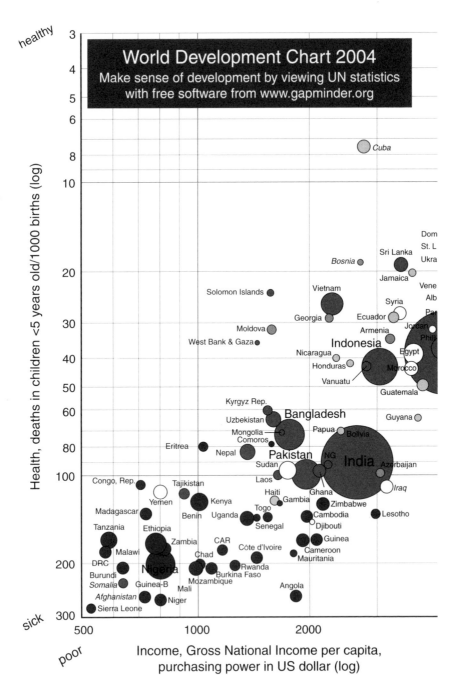

Figure 1.1: World development chart. Source: UNCDB, 2004

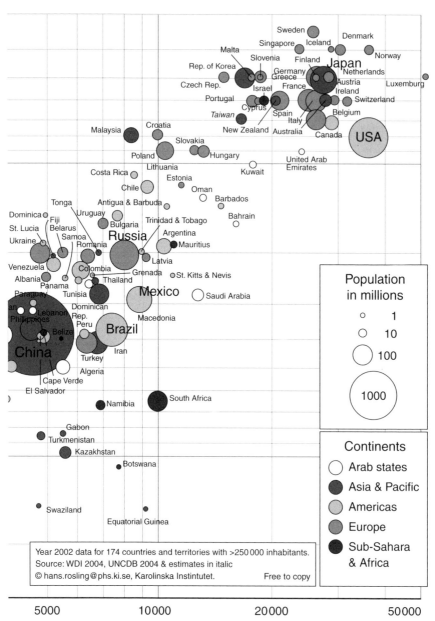

Sweden Denmark
Singapore Iceland
Malta Norway
Slovenia Finland Japan
Rep. of Korea Germany Netherlands
Greece Austria Luxemburg
Czech Rep. Israel France Ireland
Portugal Switzerland
Taiwan Cyprus Spain Belgium
Italy
New Zealand Australia Canada
Malaysia Croatia
Slovakia USA
Poland Hungary
Lithuania United Arab
Costa Rica Kuwait Emirates
Chile Estonia
Oman Barbados
Tonga Antigua & Barbuda
Dominica Uruguay Bahrain
Fiji Trinidad & Tobago
St. Lucia Belarus Bulgaria
Ukraine Samoa Argentina
Romania Russia Mauritius
Latvia
Venezuela Colombia
Albania Grenada St. Kitts & Nevis
Panama Thailand
Paraguay Tunisia Mexico Saudi Arabia
Dominican
Lebanon Rep.
Philippines Peru Macedonia
Belize Brazil
China Iran
Turkey
Algeria
Cape Verde
El Salvador
Namibia South Africa
Gabon
Turkmenistan
Kazakhstan
Botswana
Swaziland
Equatorial Guinea

Population
in millions

○   1
○   10
○   100

○ 1000

Continents
○ Arab states
● Asia & Pacific
● Americas
● Europe
● Sub-Sahara
& Africa

Year 2002 data for 174 countries and territories with >250 000 inhabitants.
Source: WDI 2004, UNCDB 2004 & estimates in italic
© hans.rosling@phs.ki.se, Karolinska Instintutet.   Free to copy

5000   10000   20000   50000

Income, Gross National Income per capita,
purchasing power in US dollar (log)

deaths of infants below the age of five years out of every 1000 born alive. The data have been graphed on log–log paper so that the relationship is rendered more clear for the lay person. One would not expect the relationship to be perfect (a nice straight line running diagonally across the page from a low point on the left to a high point on the right) because of other variables affecting health. For instance, Botswana and Russia are of approximately equal wealth, yet differ greatly in health status. But on the log–log graph most countries cluster approximately on a straight line, very roughly of equation:

$$8y = 6x + 1$$

It cannot be more exact than that without calculating from the original data before it was expressed logarithmically. In Figure 1.1, it works out approximately that for each US $1000 more in income, there is one death less.

With a graph illustrating the generally obvious, we would learn more, perhaps, by looking at the nations and territories that fall far off the expected line, either above it or below it. For instance, such a procedure might well lead us to ask why, say, Equatorial Guinea is so comparatively wealthy, yet so unhealthy? But even a cursory glance at Figure 1.1 shows one country that is so far off the expected line that it appears as though the wealth–health relationship does not apply to it. That country is Cuba. It is small and relatively poor, and yet its health status is slightly better than that of the USA. In health terms it is up there with the first-world countries. Since we are interested in finding ways of creating global equity in human rights, Cuba might well be telling us something we need to know. This issue is alluded to in the final chapter of the book.

The health–wealth problem

The latest (2004) UN classification designates five categories, as follows, in descending order of GNP:

1 High income nations.
2 Upper middle income nations.
3 Lower middle income nations.
4 Other low income nations.
5 Least developed nations.

Of course, using measures such as GNP, we can show how much money wealth actually remains in a country but, as indicated in the Preface, that is more a measure of how much money the first-world corporations leave behind after they take their profits away. Remember, Ken Sara Wiwa was murdered for asking where Nigeria's oil profits had gone. By his reckoning, Nigeria was a rich country but was not allowed to sell its own oil.

The situation on the ground, so to speak, is that, through the globalisation of the US dollar, Category 1 nations are in a dominant fiscal relationship over nations in categories 2–5. For the sake of convenience – and in keeping with current general usage – Category 1 will be designated as the 'first world' and all the others as 'third world'. More than 80% of the world's population lives in nations in categories 3–5.

The link between health and wealth is shown unambiguously in Figure 1.2.

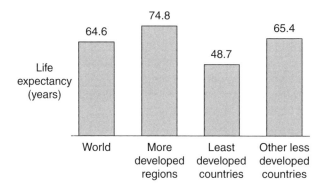

Figure 1.2: Life expectancy at birth. More developed regions: according to the United Nations (UN) Population Division these include Australia, Europe, Japan and North America. Less developed regions include Africa, Asia (excluding Japan) and Latin America and the Caribbean; 49 countries within these regions are classified as least developed. (Source: UN Population Division (2003) *World Population Prospects, 2002 revision.*)

Let us look at another breakdown, which exhibits the connection even more strongly (Table 1.1).

The proportion of a community's money that can be devoted to healthcare obviously depends on the amount available to that community altogether. But only 11% of health spending globally is made available to the 80% of the world's population living in the third

Table 1.1:   Health spending per capita by country income level 1997

Income group	Total spending on health per person (US $)
Least developed countries	11
Other low income countries (per capita GNP <US $760 in 1998)	23
Lower middle income countries (per capita GNP between US $761 and US $3030 in 1998)	93
Upper middle income countries (per capita GNP between US $3031 and US $9360 in 1998)	241
High income countries (per capita GNP >US $9360 in 1998)	1907

world. These same countries account for 90% of world disease in total (WHO, 2000).

The WHO report cited above (WHO, 2000) goes on to point out that, in third-world nations, spending on healthcare is only about US $11 per *year*. This falls far below the US $35 or so stated by the WHO as the minimum level of spending required if it is also to cover a minimal level of healthcare. Compare that with the US $2000 used yearly per person for healthcare in the first world.

It is also a fact that the common diseases which almost exclusively afflict the poorest countries attract much less research funding and professional interest than do high-profile diseases in the first world. The levels of spending in each case are largely determined by market forces, especially with regard to pharmaceuticals. Anderson *et al.* (1996) have shown that annual global research spending on malaria in 1990 was only US $65 per fatality caused by the disease, as opposed to US $789 per fatality attributed to asthma. In the four years 1975–1979, only 13 of the 1233 drugs that were available to the global market were directed at tropical infectious diseases of greatest concern to the poverty-stricken third world, according to the Global Forum for Health Research (2002).

During the last five years, initiatives such as the 'Global Alliance for Vaccines and Immunisation' have been active in trying to counter this imbalance. They have been successful in stimulating more research, and even development in the field, on diseases affecting very poor nations. Notwithstanding such successes, the Global Forum for Health

Research (2002) asserts that only a small part of research and development spending is directed at diseases accounting for 90% of the world's health problems.

It goes without saying that people living in the third world must have significantly less access to modern medical technology than those in the first. In passing, consider the impact of HIV/AIDS. In the first world anti-retroviral drugs are easily accessible. They are produced by the prominent pharmaceutical corporations at a cost far in excess of what the citizens of poor countries can routinely be expected to pay. As we know, some of the larger third-world countries, such as South Africa, India and Brazil, have developed generic copies of these anti-retroviral agents. For some years these have been regarded as medically less efficacious than the commercial brands, but, in June 1994, *The Lancet* published an article to the effect that there was no significant difference in efficacy between generic and commercial anti-retroviral drugs (Asamoah-Odei, 2004). But, as a result of this legacy of inequity, AIDS-related mortality rates are soaring in Africa. At the July 2004 meeting of the 15th International AIDS Conference, held in Bangkok, Kofi Annan commented that HIV/AIDS has now also gained a strong foothold in Asia, although not yet nearly as much as in some African nations. Particular attention is focused on this condition in Chapter 5. Suffice to say at this point, the impact of HIV/AIDS has already been such that average life expectancy is falling in a number of third-world nations (Lamptey *et al.*, 2002). In the seven African countries of Angola, Botswana, Malawi, Mozambique, Rwanda, Zambia and Zimbabwe, average life expectancy has declined to 40 years and less.

With respect to the research by Asamoah-Odei (2004), it is interesting to note that only a few weeks earlier the *British Medical Journal* carried an article by Fiona Fleck (26 June 2003) to the effect that nearly a year earlier, the WHO had withdrawn two generic AIDS drugs from its approval list. In September 2003, Fleck had revealed that the WTO had – after eight months of stalling by the US delegation – finally agreed to give poor nations access to these drugs.

TRIPS

An acronym that occurs often in such discussions is 'TRIPS' (Trade-Related Intellectual Property Rights). The above account of the generic AIDS drugs exemplifies the concept. The expensive pharmaceutical anti-retroviral agents (ARVs) are, of course, patented. Attempts by desperate third-world scientists to create cheaper, domestically produced replacements would constitute a criminal offence if they attempted to sell the drugs. But, can the poor in the third world be held to ransom by such legislation? The argument continues, and the WTO tries to impose it through its own regulations. Similar examples of this rapacious application of TRIPS against the third-world poor, to the advantage of the rich in the first world, have become legion since 2002.

Take genetically modified (GM) crops, for example. People tend to get caught up in concerns about their safety. But that is not the urgent issue. Since humankind has been growing crops, they have been genetically modifying food. Would Sir Walter Raleigh (1552–1618) even recognise a potato today as being the first of a series of genetic modifications of the tiny things he first brought to Europe? To produce GM foods, resistant to various pests, in the third world could represent a breakthrough for equity and health.

But if a particular GM crop is patented, as most are, and this patent is used (through TRIPS) as a means of preventing the third world routine access to them, it is a question of justice – a political rather than a scientific question. Even worse is the moral problem raised by large US corporations, such as Monsanto, patenting crops that are seedless. The third-world farmer can use these to produce a magnificent yield of disease-free crops. But without being able to collect seeds for the next year's crop he is stopped in his tracks. The seeds are only available by purchase from the patent-holder – once more rendering third-world health hostage to first-world wealth.

WHO and TRIPS

At the 56th World Health Assembly, organised by the WHO at Geneva in May 2000, TRIPS centred pivotally in the debate, as delegates argued about the appropriate response to the 'Report by the Secretariat on Intellectual Property Rights, Innovation and Public Health'.

Developed countries, and in particular the USA, did not want the WHO to take an aggressive approach to international property rights issues. In contrast, developing countries pushed for the delineation of a clearer role for the WHO in evaluating the public health implications of increasing intellectual property rights protection in accordance with the agreement on TRIPS, as well as under regional and bilateral trade agreements.

Furthermore, while the USA focused on prevention and health promotion, many developing countries, such as China, Brazil and Cuba, wanted the WHO to prioritise treatment and provide assistance to countries as necessary to ensure access for all to essential medicines. Brazil emphasised the significance of human rights in the fight against HIV/AIDS by producing generic copies of ARVs and exporting them cheaply to other third-world countries which required them.

The USA submitted a proposal that focused exclusively on the expression of intellectual property rights as the vehicle by which to spur innovation, and failed to make reference to the Doha Declaration* on the TRIPS agreement and public health (WTO, 2001). A coalition of non-governmental organisations, including Médecins Sans Frontières, the Treatment Action Campaign, OXFAM and the Canadian HIV/ AIDS Legal Network, responded to the USA's proposal, disputing the link between intellectual property protection and research and development, particularly into diseases that primarily affect developing countries, and pointing out the obvious role that intellectual property protection plays in creating barriers to accessing existing medicines through higher drug prices and weakened generic competition.

A strong pro-health resolution that incorporated developing country concerns was brought to the table by Brazil and later co-sponsored by Bolivia, Ecuador, Indonesia, Peru, Venezuela and South Africa, on behalf of the members of the WHO African Region. The resolution advocated a clear mandate for the WHO to monitor the impact of TRIPS, as well as bilateral and regional agreements on public health and innovation, and also called for the creation of an independent commission similar to the United Kingdom Commission on Intellectual Property Rights. Extensive consultations between Brazil, the USA and a number of African delegations led to the adoption of a compromise text in the final resolution on 'Intellectual Property Rights, Innovation and Public Health'. Included is a request for the establishment of a time-limited body to investigate appropriate funding and incentive methods for the development of new medicines for 'neglected diseases' as well as a request for WHO co-operation at the invitation of a member state to develop 'pharmaceutical and health policies and

---

*Item 17 of the Doha Declaration states that the TRIPS agreement must always be interpreted in a manner supportive of public health. This should obviously apply to the freedom to produce more accessible ARVs generically.

regulatory measures' to 'mitigate the negative impacts' of international trade agreements. The non-governmental organisations expressed some disappointment with the final text of the resolution, as well as the exclusion of the text proposed by China that would have reaffirmed the primacy of health over trade concerns and acknowledged the difficulties developing countries face in making use of compulsory licensing as provided for in the Doha Declaration.

Is this a case of, once again, trade rights having priority over health rights? Is this yet another example of a new and more efficient continuation of first-world imperialism over the third?

The problem of global variations in health

In order to address the issue of making primary healthcare available to all as a right, we need to consider the vexing problems posed because great disparities of health exist between, and even within, geographic territories across the globe. Even within first-world countries such as the UK and the USA there are variations in health. These variations are particularly acute in the USA, where about 32% of the population is unable to afford health insurance and where 'Medicare' and 'Medicaid'* provision varies from state to state. Even in first-world nations such as Finland, Holland and the UK the poor die about seven or eight years before the rich. And that is in countries in which all citizens have access to healthcare. Such apparent anomalies can, to a great extent, be accounted for by the fact that poorer people are more likely to seek out pre-cooked meals because they lack the income for good kitchen facilities. They are likely to smoke more and to drink more. They also live in less safe areas of large cities. For instance, in the London borough of Newham (one of the poorest boroughs in the UK), a primary school child is six times more likely to be run over than is the case in the London borough of Richmond-upon-Thames. In the latter, of course, there are far more parks and play areas that are safe from road traffic (Doran, 2000).

Similarly, there is within-country variation in access to healthcare within the poorest countries of the world. But if we look at the diseases that contribute most to the between-community discrepancies in health, we find that the most common are various tropical parasitic

---

* In the USA, Medicaid is a publicly funded scheme that provides part of the medical costs of people below a certain income level. Medicare is a similar scheme for the elderly.

diseases, such as malaria, and diseases like HIV/AIDS, which depend on widespread lack of education and human rights, and on lack of access to pharmaceutical prophylactic agents for their spread and their impact.

In the third world, and especially among the poorest populations, many of the standard measures of wealth or poverty are not applicable. The 'Demographic and Health Survey' (DHS) programme, originally set up in Latin America in the early 1990s, is now proving to be one of the most powerful measures of health status in the third world ever devised. It is a survey research project which is being carried out in Africa, Asia and Latin America. Arising from pilot studies, the DHS is based on measures such as the ownership of (or access to) a refrigerator, television and radio; possession of a car, motorcycle or bicycle; how the household dwelling is constructed and from which materials; the dwelling's source of drinking water; how toilet facilities are mediated; as well as the employment of domestic staff. Obviously, some of the index criteria, such as access to drinking water, for example, are also direct criteria for health status (Skidmore, 2002).

The household wealth index, used in the study of the DHS criteria mentioned above, allows researchers to determine a country-specific or relative definition of economic status, rather than an absolute definition. The population of each country is divided into five income groups or quintiles, calculated on the basis of their relative standing on the household wealth index within each country involved. For example, the economic status of the lowest quintile in Haiti would not be at all similar to that of the poorest quintile in Argentina (World Bank, 2003).

Economists engaged in such studies of global research often use an 'absolute' or 'universal' measure of poverty. Such an approach tries to define poverty in terms of a minimal level of income, or of consumption that is universally applicable and fixed in time. The reader can appreciate the difficulties involved. It would work somewhat as follows. Researchers would estimate the minimal amount of money required for food and other essentials across the countries concerned. Consideration of what level of nutrition is to be taken as basic or of what constitutes 'other essentials' are the subject of much analysis and argument.

During 2001–2002, the World Bank (2003) calculated that the 'international' or 'absolute' poverty line was approximately US $1 per day average income, but even this figure had to be statistically adjusted for variations in purchasing power between countries. In the author's experience, gained while working in communities where such discussions are not academic, the sheer obscenity of real people living out their lives like this is overwhelming.

The World Bank estimated, in 2002, that 1.2 billion people were living (surviving!) on less than US $1 a day. The bank points out that this represents progress because the figure is down from 1.3 billion people (a difference of 100 million) in 1990. However, the author calculated – using the same sources – that over the same period there was an increase in the number of people living on less than US $2 a day. That is, money was being transferred from the already desperately poor to those who were even more desperately poor! Any kind of equitable global wealth aid system would shift the money easily from the first world to the third world to remove both obscenities. Doing so would have a negligible effect on citizens in the first world, and have an enormous impact on the health of people in the third world.

Measures such as levels of education, existing health status, languages used and foreign languages known* and living conditions can be used as crude estimates for determining economic well-being. Such measures can draw attention to aspects of poverty that would otherwise escape notice. In other words, we need to become far more conscious of 'types' of poverty. This will involve going further than using standard measures of income and consumption to allow us to ascertain levels of poverty and their impact on health.

'The World Bank once viewed poverty as largely income-based, but now we see it as multidimensional' (Quesada, 2003). Much of this change in emphasis may be attributed to the germinal insights of Amartya Sen, who, in 1998, won the Nobel Prize in Economics. Specifically, he objected to the conventional ways of measuring poverty, based on working out the proportion of populations whose incomes fell below some 'poverty line'. Amartya Sen is quoted as saying, 'You cannot draw a poverty line and then apply it across the board to everyone in the same way, without taking into account personal characteristics and circumstances.' What Sen advocated was that poverty analysis needs to focus on people's access to opportunities

---

*You only need to work in the third world to realise that people who share their native language with millions of others are in a far stronger position of health empowerment than are people whose languages only embrace comparatively small numbers. To even be only moderately fluent in a metropolitan language, such as English, Spanish, Chinese or Arabic, can have an enormous impact on health and opportunities in general.

(profoundly affected by native language, in this author's view) in health and education as well as their social capabilities (Mach, 2003).

Within-poor-community variation

The author has already referred to the 'within'-community variations in health in wealthy countries such as the UK and the USA. Lessons to be learnt from this variation include the sobering realisation that domestic health legislation cannot alone level the playing field, much to the chagrin of social democratic thinkers. For instance, the inception of the NHS in the UK in 1948 was hailed as a brilliant triumph for socialist (Labour Party) health legislation. The author recalls it being referred to by a Marxist–Leninist lecturer in Czechoslovakia at the time as, 'so good it will be even as good as the Soviet Union', as he excitedly translated from an editorial in the English-language *Manchester Guardian* (MacDonald, 2005). As we know from the Black Report (Townsend and Davidson, 1982) and other findings, huge (and increasing) gaps in health status within the population prevail, despite an NHS that confers treatment without cost to the patient. In the USA there is no equivalent to the NHS, so the same situation is less unexpected.

But what happens in the third world, in which government healthcare is patchy or – more commonly – non-existent? Let us look at a number of dimensions of health status, as discussed earlier. Care-seeking behaviour, diagnosis and treatment, along with disease incidence and mortality rates, are all measures that are inextricably wealth-dependent. DHS data provided the basis for a huge multi-country study covering the 12-year period from 1990 to 2002. It showed poor/non-poor differences in health status and use made of existing health services across a whole gamut of reproductive health indicators. Table 1.2 shows the country-by-country results (Gwatkin and Davidson, 2003). As well as that, other multi-country studies have demonstrated statistically significant relationships between health and economic status.

Table 1.2: Poor–non-poor inequalities in health – selected indicators

Country	Under-5 mortality rate (deaths of children under 5 per 1000 live births)		Malnutrition among women/ mothers (% with Body Mass Index* < 18.6 kg/m²)*		Children aged 12 months to 23 months who were fully vaccinated (%)		Women receiving delivery assistance from a doctor or nurse/midwife (%)	
	Poorest quintile	Richest quintile	Poorest quintile	Richest quintile	Poorest quintile	Richest quintile	Poorest quintile	Richest quintile
East Asia, Pacific								
Cambodia, 2000	155	64	24	17	29	68	15	81
Indonesia, 1997	109	29	–	–	43	72	21	89
Philippines, 1998	80	29	–	–	60	87	21	92
Vietnam, 1997	63	23	–	–	42	60	49	99
Vietnam, 2000	53	16	–	–	44	92	58	100
Europe, Central Asia								
Armenia, 2000	61	30	3	4	66	(68)	93	100
Kazakhstan, 1995	48	40	11	7	21	(34)	99	100
Kazakhstan, 1999	82	45	7	9	69	(62)	99	99
Kyrgyz Republic, 1997	96	49	7	7	69	73	96	100
Turkey, 1993	125	27	3	3	41	82	43	99
Turkey, 1998	85	33	2	2	28	70	53	98
Turkmenistan, 2000	106	70	11	10	86	89	97	98
Uzbekistan, 1996	70	50	12	8	81	78	92	100
Latin America and the Caribbean								
Bolivia, 1998	147	32	0.5	2	22	31	20	98
Brazil, 1996	99	33	9	5	57	74	72	99
Colombia, 1995	52	24	6	1	58	77	61	98
Colombia, 2000	39	20	3	3	50	65	64	99
Dominican Republic, 1996	90	27	10	6	34	47	89	98
Guatemala, 1995	89	38	4	2	49	46	9	92
Guatemala, 1998	78	39	4	0.5	66	56	9	92
Haiti, 1994–1995	163	106	25	9	19	44	2	65
Haiti, 2000	164	109	17	8	25	42	4	70
Nicaragua, 1997–1998	69	30	4	4	61	73	33	92
Nicaragua, 2001	64	19	3	4	64	71	78	99
Paraguay, 1990	57	20	–	–	20	53	41	98
Peru, 1996	110	22	1	1	55	66	14	97
Peru, 2000	93	18	1	2	58	81	13	88

Table 1.2:   Continued

Middle East/North Africa								
Egypt, 1995	147	39	–	–	65	93	21	86
Egypt, 2000	98	34	1	0.1	91	92	31	94
Jordan, 1997	42	25	3	2	21	17	91	99
Morocco, 1992	112	39	6	2	54	95	5	78
Yemen, 1997	163	73	39	13	8	56	7	50
South Asia								
Bangladesh, 1996–1997	141	76	65	33	47	67	2	30
Bangladesh, 1999–2000	140	72	–	–	50	75	4	42
India, 1992–1993	155	54	–	–	17	65	12	79
India, 1998–1999	141	46	50	15	21	64	16	84
Nepal, 1996	156	83	26	21	32	71	3	34
Nepal, 2001	130	68	27	15	54	82	4	45
Pakistan, 1990–1991	125	74	–	–	23	55	5	55
Sub-Saharan Africa								
Benin, 1996	208	110	21	7	38	74	34	98
Benin, 2001	198	93	16	6	49	73	50	99
Burkina Faso, 1998–1999	239	155	16	9	21	52	18	75
Cameroon, 1991	201	82	–	–	27	64	32	95
Cameroon, 1998	199	87	12	4	24	57	28	89
Central African Republic, 1994–1995	193	98	16	11	18	64	14	82
Chad, 1996–1997	171	172	28	21	4	23	3	47
Comoros, 1996	129	(87)	7	9	40	82	26	85
Côte d'Ivoire, 1994	194	97	11	6	16	64	17	84
Eritrea, 1995	152	104	45	21	25	84	5	74
Ethiopia, 2000	159	147	32	25	7	34	0.9	25
Gabon, 2000	93	55	9	4	6	24	67	97
Ghana, 1993	156	75	12	7	38	79	25	85
Ghana, 1998	139	52	18	5	50	79	18	86
Guinea, 1999	230	133	17	9	17	52	12	82
Kenya, 1998	136	61	18	6	48	60	23	80
Madagascar, 1997	195	101	24	15	22	66	30	89
Malawi, 1992	253	172	14	6	73	89	45	78
Malawi, 2000	231	149	10	6	65	81	43	83
Mali, 1995–1996	298	169	16	12	16	56	11	81
Mali, 2001	248	148	13	10	20	56	8	82

Table 1.2: Continued

Country	Under-5 mortality rate (deaths of children under 5 per 1000 live births)		Malnutrition among women/ mothers (% with Body Mass Index* < 18.6 kg/m²)*		Children aged 12 months to 23 months who were fully vaccinated (%)		Women receiving delivery assistance from a doctor or nurse/midwife (%)	
	Poorest quintile	Richest quintile	Poorest quintile	Richest quintile	Poorest quintile	Richest quintile	Poorest quintile	Richest quintile
Mauritania, 2000–2001	98	79	17	9	16	45	15	93
Mozambique, 1997	278	145	17	4	20	85	18	82
Namibia, 1992	110	76	19	5	54	63	51	91
Namibia, 2000	55	31	–	–	60	68	55	97
Niger, 1998	282	184	27	13	5	51	4	63
Nigeria, 1990	240	120	–	–	14	58	12	70
Rwanda, 2000	146	154	12	7	71	79	17	60
Senegal, 1997	181	70	–	–	–	–	20	86
South Africa, 1998	87	22	–	–	51	70	68	98
Tanzania, 1996	140	98	12	7	57	83	27	81
Tanzania, 1999	160	135	–	–	53	78	29	83
Togo, 1998	168	97	13	8	22	52	25	91
Uganda, 1995	192	113	13	6	34	63	23	70
Uganda, 2000–2001	192	106	15	5	27	32	20	77
Zambia, 1996	212	136	10	8	71	86	19	91
Zambia, 2001–2002	192	92	21	10	64	80	20	91
Zimbabwe, 1994	85	56	6	1	72	86	55	93
Zimbabwe, 1999	100	62	9	4	64	64	57	94

Note: Figures have been rounded.
* Body Mass Index is based on weight in kilograms divided by square of height in metres. In some countries, surveys measured malnutrition among women ages 15 to 49 or 15 to 44; in other countries, the surveys measured malnutrition among women with children under 5 years of age.
( ) Parentheses indicate that the figure is based on a relatively small number of cases and may not be reliable.
Source: Gwatkin and Davidson, 2003
dash = data not available

References

Anderson J et al. (1996) Malaria Research: an audit of international activity. PRISM Report 7. The Wellcome Trust, Unit for Policy Research in Science and Medicine, London.

Asamoah-Odei E (2004) HIV prevalence trends in sub-Saharan Africa – no decline and large sub-regional differences. The Lancet. 364: 35–40.

Dodgson C (1983) Alice in Wonderland. Grosset & Dunlap, New York, NY.

Doran E (2000) *Newham Health Improvement Program: Road Safety Program, NHS Newham Trust.* HMSO, London.

Fleck F (2003) World Trade Organization finally agrees to cheap drugs deal. *BMJ.* **327**: 517.

Global Forum for Health Research (2002) *Report on Health Research 2001–2002.* World Health Organization, Geneva.

Gwatkin D and Davidson R (2003) *Initial Country-level Information about Socio-economic Differences in Health, Nutrition and Population.* Karolinska Institutet, Stockholm.

Lamptey P, Wigley M, Carr D and Collymore Y (2002) *Facing the HIV/AIDS Pandemic.* Population Reference Bureau, Washington, DC.

MacDonald T (2005) *Third World Health: hostage to first world wealth.* Radcliffe Publishing, Oxford.

Mach A (2003) Amartya Sen on development and health: 'To Our Health'. www.who.int/infwha52/to-our-health/amartya.html. Accessed 2 September 2005.

Matthiason N and Townsend M (2005) Campaign: countdown to G8. *Observer.* 15 May.

Quesada C (2003) Amartya Sen and the thousand faces of poverty. International Development Bank (IDB) America. www.ladb.org. Accessed 9 August 2005.

Sanders D (2005) Primary Healthcare and Health System Development: Strategies for Revitalisation. Paper presented to the People's Health Assembly, July, Ecuador.

Skidmore P (2002) *Demographic and Health Survey Dimensions No. 4.* HMSO, London.

Townsend P and Davidson N (1982) *Inequalities in Health: The Black Report.* Penguin, London.

UN Population Division (2003) *World Population Prospects: the 2002 revision.* UN Population Division, New York, NY.

UNCDB (2004) *World Development Chart.* Division of International Health, Department of Public Health Sciences, Karolinska Institutet, Stockholm.

World Bank (2003) *World Development Indicators.* World Bank, Washington, DC.

World Health Organization (1973) *Organizational Study on Methods of Promoting the Development of Basic Health Services.* Annex 11, Official WHO Records No. 26. WHO, Geneva.

World Health Organization (1978) *The Alma Ata Declaration – HFA (2000).* World Health Assembly, Geneva.

World Health Organization (2000) *The World Health Report.* WHO, Geneva.

World Trade Organization (2001) Doha Declaration on TRIPS and Health – 4th Ministerial Council Declaration. www.wto.org. Accessed 9 August 2005.

Chapter 2

First-world finance: third-world poverty

A brief conspectus of development

One of the greatest presidents that the USA ever had was Franklin Delano Roosevelt (1882–1945). To many Americans he is still remembered with almost reverential affection, for, whilst the aftermath of the Great Depression was causing immense suffering to working people across the USA, he introduced the New Deal, with its vast relief programmes and assistance to industry and agriculture. Franklin D Roosevelt was indeed a remarkable man, American (in the best possible sense of that word) to the core and committed to the welfare of his people. At the age of 39 he was severely crippled by polio, but that did not stop him from becoming President in 1933 and from being re-elected in 1936, 1940 and 1944.

One measure of Roosevelt's credentials as an American was reflected in his devotion to the idea of 'the common people' and his parallel dislike of royalty or anything that smacked of privilege by wealth or social class. For that reason, he felt an intense animus toward the British Empire, whose preferential tariff and trade arrangements with its colonies and dominions effectively hindered the USA in its attempts to enhance its own overseas trade. Therefore, on coming to office in 1933, he was determined to dismantle the British Empire and to promote American trading interests. Although many third-world people may well have lauded the first of those aims, they have since paid heavily for the success of the second.

It was in this context that Roosevelt, along with the famous English economist, John Maynard Keynes (1883–1946), played such a pivotal role in setting up the three major financial bodies which today control the levers of global trade. These bodies are the World Bank (officially known as the International Bank for Reconstruction and Development), the International Monetary Fund (IMF) and – somewhat later – the World Trade Organization (WTO). Now closely associated with these organisations are financial agreements such as the General Agreement on Tariffs and Trade (GATT), the General Agreement on Trade in Services (GATS) and various bilateral and free trade linkages such as the North America Free Trade Agreement (NAFTA) (Shoup and Mintel, 1977).

GATT was set up in 1948 to try to rationalise international trade, especially trade between the USA and other countries. But the enterprise was bedevilled by immense administrative difficulties and lacked strong leadership. During its 47-year history, GATT policy-making meetings have been held in Havana (Cuba), Annecy (France), Torquay (the UK), Tokyo (Japan), Punta del Este (Uruguay), Montreal (Canada), Brussels (Belgium) and, lastly, Marrakesh (Morocco) in 1994. During that period, the entire trading system came under GATT after a failed attempt to set up another overarching body, the Industrial Trade Organization (ITO). The third world was not significantly consulted in this activity but has since been deeply affected by it, for it represented the first attempt to systematically organise globalised finance under a neo-liberal orthodoxy.

In 1995, GATT was replaced by the WTO, a much more tightly organised body, with a governing General Council and powers to arbitrate in trade disputes between member nations. For instance, in July 2005, the WTO Council ruled the European Union (EU) out of order in the latter's attempts to protect small, individually owned banana plantations in tiny Caribbean island nations such as St Lucia. The ruling, in effect, gives Chiquita – the large South American banana-producing multi-national (largely owned by US stockholders) – all the rights to free trade in bananas with EU states.

GATS represented an even broader application of neo-liberal economics, extending its remit to services such as healthcare and education. In fact, GATS can be said to have truly designated health as a tradeable commodity rather than a basic human right. GATS came into being at the WTO General Council meeting in Cancun, Mexico, in September 2003. There is natural concern that promises made by the EU and the USA in other WTO discussions will be used to extract further services liberalisation (such as the privatisation of healthcare) under GATS. Basically, then, GATS has been an international trade agreement since 1995 and is under the control of the WTO. Its objective is to remove all barriers to global trade in both goods and services. With respect to the latter, it covers both health and education. The idea is to open these services up to international competition, allowing large for-profit multi-national firms to compete with domestic services. In 1999, the European Commission actually stated, 'The GATS is not just something that exists between governments. It is first and foremost an instrument for the benefit of business' (GATS Watch, 2005).

Since February 2000, negotiations have been underway in the WTO to expand and 'fine tune' the GATS. These negotiations have aroused widespread concern in the third world. A growing number of local governments, trade unions, non-governmental organisations, governments of small countries and so forth are criticising these talks and calling for them to end. Their main concerns are that they will result in:

- negative effects on universal access to safe water, transport and basic health, and education provision
- restrictions on the rights of local governments to control and mediate international companies in areas such as tourism, tele-communications, the media and so on
- preventing prior assessment by local governments of the potential impact of overseas-financed groups on such activities
- the destruction of domestically accountable infrastructures and services.

The effect of neo-liberalism on primary healthcare

It is worthwhile to examine the impact of neoliberal policies on primary healthcare. We will start with a common enough health measure used by epidemiologists: infant mortality rates. Infant mortality rate is defined as the number of babies who die in their first year of life, of each 1000 live births. From 1961 to 1980, the decrease in infant mortality rates worldwide was 38.5. Even in sub-Saharan Africa (to cite one particularly poor region) there was a decline of 19.2/1000 live births. From 1980 to 1999, the rate of decline slowed considerably to 27 worldwide and to only 15 in sub-Saharan Africa (UNICEF, 2000). Over the period from 1950 to 1995, life expectancy rose from 46 years to 65 years worldwide, while the number of children under five years of age who died out of every 1000 born alive dropped from 17.5 million to 10.5 million per year.

These radical improvements came about mainly because of exten-sive community campaigns to monitor polio, diphtheria and other

controllable illnesses through immunisation and other control programmes, but since then there has been a large-scale reversal of past
gains because of the imposition of various IMF-approved strategies to
render healthcare self-financing (UNICEF, 2003).

During these latter years, neo-liberal globalisation has resulted in
inequitable access to funding for community health programmes. It
has seen, for instance, programmes for HIV/AIDS treatment become
dependent on individuals having to pay for ARVs. Under present
WTO rules, such treatments are relentlessly becoming available only
from multi-national pharmaceutical firms at a cost well beyond most
people's means in the third world. In fact, World Bank structural
adjustment policies have led to:

- cuts in expenditure on government-funded health programmes
- the introduction of various 'cost-recovery' modalities, by which
  communities and individuals are pressured to make a financial
  contribution for services
- devaluation of the local currency to meet trade adjustments
- free trade in food staples, impoverishing local farmers.

Financial and trade globalisation under WTO control has liberalised
trade and thus allowed trans-national corporations to overwhelm
domestic markets. Henry Kissinger, American Secretary of State
(1973–1977) under presidents Nixon and Ford, said in a public lecture
in Dublin on 12 October 1999:

> *The process of development begins by widening the gap between the
> rich and the poor in each country. ... The basic challenge is that what
> is called globalisation is really none other than the name given to the
> dominant role of the United States.*

The matter could hardly have been stated more forcefully had it been
made by a primary healthcare field worker hostile to the process. But
the figures are far more persuasively eloquent. During 1960–1962 the
Gross Domestic Product (GDP) of the poorest and richest countries,
respectively, were US $212 and US $11 474. But that was before the
neo-liberal globalisation of finance got a grip. The corresponding
figures for 2002–2003 were US $267 and US $32 339, respectively
(Sanders, 2005).

Origins of the present trading systems

From 1942 onwards, the USA and the UK collaborated, through a series of meetings at Bretton Woods, to draw up plans for financing international free trade. The key British delegate in this was none other than John Maynard Keynes. By 1944, the idea of two separate agencies had gelled: the International Bank for Reconstruction and Development, now called the World Bank, and the International Monetary Fund (IMF), but with different functions. Keynes suggested setting up a world trade organisation then as well, but this idea was rejected by Roosevelt as not being in the interests of US trade. The WTO was set up in 1995 when it became clear that US interests could be well served by it.

The IMF agrees on broad lines of policy in matters such as establishing and maintaining currency convertibility, and avoiding competitive exchange depreciation. Thus, unlike the World Bank, it was set up as a think-tank and not only as a financial institution. Its basic financial policy was initially to adhere strictly to the gold standard in adjudicating loans to member countries. However, the USA came off the gold standard in the early 1960s. Thus the IMF was restrained from high-risk lending. Indeed, it only lends to treasuries and central banks of member countries, and generally over only five years. The IMF sees its function as to help its members in the short term should they run into balance-of-payments problems (Rachman and Bloch, 1974).

The World Bank has virtually the same membership as the IMF, but has much more financial flexibility. For instance, it can make long-term loans over periods like 20 years and can now lend to private projects in third-world countries. In this way it can directly influence the running of those countries. The World Bank makes wide use of private banks in the first and third world as principal and intermediary lenders. It can also sell outstanding debts on the financial markets. Indeed, it is this capacity of first-world bankers to 'sell outstanding debts' that keeps them safe, while mortgaging the third world still further.

Structural adjustment

The most visual impact that the IMF and World Bank policies have had on third world health relates to what the World Bank called 'structural adjustment', which it began to demand of borrower nations in the late 1970s. In fact, there is a considerable body of opinion that it was this imposition that played a major role in precipitating the so-called 'debt crisis' of the 1980s.

In order to try to reduce the risks involved in lending money to third-world countries, the World Bank began to consider the possibility of making its loans conditional on the government of the debtor nation implementing certain changes to its current spending policies. Generally these 'structural adjustments' involved having to move money away from the public sector to the private one. They also involved a switch in healthcare and education policies, from 'horizontalisation' to 'verticalisation'. The 'debt crisis' of the early 1980s is easily seen to link with structural adjustment policies as well.

Very briefly, the debt crisis arose suddenly, and in roughly the following manner. In the late 1970s, the oil-producing nations agreed to raise their prices dramatically. Industrialised nations of the first world cannot do without oil and gasoline, so they had little choice but to accept the consequences of this decision. But, for poorer nations importing oil-based fuels such a price rise was catastrophic. They had to keep their factories running to produce and sell in order to obtain dollar currency to pay off their debt (IMF and World Bank loan repayments have to be in US dollars). The increasing fuel prices meant that they had to renegotiate existing debts and sometimes borrow even more.

The sequence of events behind the debt crisis

Oil (which is priced in dollars) dropped in value and, in 1973, the Organization of Petroleum Exporting Countries (OPEC) increased oil prices. This caused OPEC members to accumulate dollars, which they then deposited in first-world banks, principally in the USA. Of course, these US banks were having to pay interest on such deposits, and they found themselves with an immense amount of money that had to be lent out quickly and in volume so that – through collecting the interest on such loans – the US banks could afford to pay the interest on the OPEC members' deposits. Impoverished third-world countries represented an ideal source of borrowers, and the banks were not too fussy about to whom they lent the money, or for what purpose. We are talking about routine business transactions here, not attempts to referee human dignity and rights. The debtor nation borrowers were generally keen to get their hands on easy loans. In the main this borrowing was to pay increased oil prices but, in addition, many of the debtor nations were recently independent countries and were anxious to build up public infrastructures in areas such as healthcare and education. However, as can easily be imagined, some were nations run by relatively corrupt administrations and/or sought an infusion of money to purchase arms, for instance, or even to reinforce the power of the ruling élite against their own people. The lenders, as already indicated, were not overly concerned about this.

Loans were offered at low (but variable) interest rates, sometimes even below the rate of inflation. The banks usually assured themselves that a particular third-world borrower nation could pay back its loan by ascertaining that the country could produce some commodity, or commodities, needed in bulk by the first world, for example crops like sugar or coffee. Initially, such commodities drew high prices, but this situation changed as more and more countries found themselves in frantic competition with each other, each nation trying to produce far more, and at a greater rate then ever before, to satisfy the same markets. This brought about a collapse of markets in these commodities, a situation especially drastic for the poor nations that were tied to a one-crop economy. The worldwide recession appearing simultaneously meant that export quantities dropped. In the meantime, because the US government had so grossly overspent on defence and had to cut taxes (to stay in power), it had to increase interest rates sharply, which, of course, increased the cost of debt repayment.

In 1979, the OPEC member countries united in raising oil prices. This had a particularly severe impact on the poor third-world countries that had rapidly begun to industrialise as a means of meeting their commitments. These countries therefore increased their borrowing and negotiated extensions on existing loans. Some, indeed, entered a spiral of unrepayable debt. As reported by Christian Aid (1998), Mexico was but one country that found itself in that situation.

In 1992, UNICEF estimated that 500 000 children a week were dying as a direct result of this debt crisis (UNICEF, 1992). This is a perfect example of the mordant logic behind the comments made by the former president of Citicorp Bank about countries not passing out of existence, even if people do. In this case we are talking about people paying with their lives for debts incurred before they were born and for the benefit of others.

Some consequences of the debt crisis

Though a given debtor nation may be impoverished and/or, because of poor government, be unable to maintain an adequate programme in health and education, these aspects of its national life are often rendered even worse through obligations to the IMF and the World Bank. For instance, from 1995 to 1998, the poorest countries of Africa paid US $13 billion annually to their creditors (Christian Aid, 1998). Contrast this with the US $9 billion that UNICEF estimated was needed for health and nutrition in all Africa. Then again, in Uganda, for every dollar the government spends per person on health, it pays eight dollars per person for debt repayment to first-world creditors. According to UNICEF (1998), in the five most indebted countries:

- children are 30% less likely to live out their first year
- a pregnant woman is three times more likely to die in childbirth
- illiteracy rates are about 25% higher
- access to safe water is about 33% lower than is the case in the five least indebted countries.

We have the anomalous situation of the poor funding the rich. In 1996, the debtor nations paid US $1.8 billion more in debt service to the IMF than they received in new loans. Since 1987 the IMF has received US $2.4 billion more from Africa than it has provided in new finance. Altogether, the poorest nations in Africa had transferred US $167 billion into debt service to their creditors in the first world by the end of 2002. This transfer of resources from the poor to the rich explains why sub-Saharan Africa cannot prevent recurring famine.

Debt, environment and health

As third-world countries attempt to meet their debt repayments through invoking the structural adjustment procedures imposed by the World Bank, they tend to sacrifice their environmental endowments, and thus the health of their people. This works roughly as follows. IMF loans must be repaid in US dollars, therefore, whatever crop, say sugar, a third-world country can produce in abundance is sold to first-world markets. Other similarly endowed third-world nations, of course, do the same, thus coming into competition with one another and ultimately causing the price of the commodity to fall. To keep production at the highest possible levels, at the lowest cost, deforestation routinely occurs at a great rate. This not only results in increased levels of carbon dioxide, erosion, pollution of air and water supplies, but requires a huge infrastructure (roads, mills and so on) to be built to transport the crop from the interior to the ports. Organised labour (if it exists) has to be exploited and union rights are abolished to cut costs, so that along with health, human rights also suffer. As already noted, there is inevitably a sharp rise in greenhouse gases.

Of course, greenhouse gases can be, and always have been, produced by non-human activities, but their immense increase during the 1970s and 1980s can easily be traced to human intervention. Indeed, the third world is not even responsible for most of this. It is estimated that 70% of this accumulation is produced by the richest 25% of the world's people – it is a first-world phenomenon. But it is the sudden increase in greenhouse gas emission from the destruction of forests in the third world – very much linked with the perceived 'needs' of the world's wealthiest people – that is of concern here.

Bunyard (1985) and Myers (1989) have provided us with empirical data on the relationship between greenhouse gas emission and deforestation rates in the 1980s, but the rate of deforestation has greatly accelerated since then. Leggett (1990) argues that deforestation in the third world accounts for as much as 20% of the global climate change we are now experiencing. Perhaps the link between this and debt is best illustrated by a table derived from George's pivotal (1992) publication.

In Table 2.1 the three columns, from left to right, are to be read as follows. In the first column the top 24 third-world debtors are listed in descending order of the amounts they had been lent. The second column lists the countries that were the largest deforesters from 1980 to 1990, again in descending order. The estimates on which these rankings are based are those of Myers (1989). The third column simply indicates the percentage of forest existing in 1980, which had been destroyed by 1989.

From the figures shown in Table 2.1 a number of things should be evident to the reader. The expression 'short-term' was used in my description of the advantages of deforestation. So short-term are these advantages that, at the present rate, the forests will cease to provide this income necessary for debt repayment long before the debt can be repaid. Also, the impact of such large-scale deforestation, even in the short-term, has wholly negative effects on health promotion – both in the countries concerned and globally. Locally, forest cover is removed, wildlife destroyed, water supplies polluted (especially by

Table 2.1: Between third-world debt and third-world relationship rates of deforestation

Rank	Country (debt in US $ million)	Rank	Deforestation acc. 1980s World Resources Institute/Myers	Percentage of original forest already destroyed
1	Brazil (112.5)	1	Brazil*	23
2	Mexico (112)	2	Indonesia*	30
3	Argentina (65)	3	Myanmar	51
4	India (60)	4	Mexico*	58
5	Indonesia (53)	5	Columbia*	63
6	China (45)	6	Thailand*	83
7	South Korea (44)	7	Malaysia*	48
8	Nigeria (31)	8	India*	90
9	Venezuela (30)	9	Nigeria*	61
10	Philippines (29)	10	Zaire*	20
11	Algeria (28)	11	Papua New Guinea	15
12	Thailand (24)	12	Vietnam	77
13	Chile (22)	13	Peru*	26
14	Peru (20.7)	14	Central America*	82
15	Morocco (20.5)	15	Ecuador*	42
16	Central America (20)	16	Philippines*	80
17	Malaysia (19.5)	17	Côte d'Ivoire*	90
18	Pakistan (18)	18	Cameroon	25
19	Columbia (16.5)	19	Venezuela*	16
20	Côte d'Ivoire (14.5)	20	Madagascar	61
21	Ecuador (12.5)	21	Bolivia	22
22	Vietnam (11.6)			
23	Bangladesh (10.7)			
24	Sudan (10)			

* Member of the 'Over $10 billion' debtor club.

the superphosphates required for quick pasture production) and globally, the ozone layer is assaulted.

In much the same way, the debt crisis has fuelled the production of narcotic drugs in the third world for sale to illegal markets in the first world (*New York Times*, 2001).

Upholding the banks

If a private bank makes a 'bad' loan to a third-world country, the loan is taken over by the IMF or the World Bank, and the shareholders do not lose. In all first-world countries, such loans are protected through the tax system. If you live in a first-world society, and are not a bank stockholder, you do not get a return of the profit generated by loan repayments, but you must pay – through tax increases – if there are losses. In reality this situation is even more bizarre than that. While it is possible for an individual borrower to completely disappear and terminate payments by dying, that almost never happens to a nation, even a third-world nation. If, for example, a loan to a third-world nation goes 'bad', this rarely means that the money is lost irretrievably. What it means is that repayments are delayed – and interest is even charged on the delays – so ultimately the lending bank recovers much more than it ever lent out. Since the IMF started, few nations have yet paid off their debt to it. But even though the actual debts remain unpaid, in total the first-world banks have made back at least three times the amount they paid out (OECD, 2000). Even if the banks immediately 'forgave' all outstanding debts and folded up their tents and went home, they would have made a healthy profit on the project.

If, for any given tax year, the first-world bank had not received the full amount of scheduled debt repayment, tax on it is exonerated. The banks don't really lose because, should the amount eventually be paid up, they don't have to pay 'back tax' on it. But the effect of this is that the loss of tax to the governments is real enough and has to be made up out of everyone else's tax. Not only that, there has been a tendency since 1980 for 'bad debt' from third-world borrowers to be moved from private banks to being a government responsibility, adding to the tax burden of citizens in the first world. This is well shown by OECD figures for 1989, as represented in Table 2.2, in which the initials LDC stand for 'less developed countries' – another euphemism for the third world.

Table 2.2: Bank loans to and returns from less-developed countries debtors ($ US billion)

Year	1982	1983	1984	1985	1986	1987	1988	1989
Total LDC debt	854	937	961	1078	1194	1329	1313	1322
LDC debt owed to commercial banks	493	516	520	554	584	630	625	629
Percentage of total debt held by banks	57.7	55	54	51	49	47	47	47
LDC debt service to banks	82.2	69.7	77.9	83.6	69.3	66.5	84.5	82
New bank lending to LDCs	37.9	35	17.2	15.2	7	7	5.8	8.5
Service to banks as percentage of debt held by banks in same year	16.7	13.4	15	15	12	10.5	13.5	13

LDC = less developed countries. Source: OECD, 1990

Whatever the nationality of the people of the borrower nation (the third-world country in this case), the transaction is always in US dollars. All the private banks in the first world who are in the business of lending money to third-world nations therefore store up US dollars. When these are passed over, therefore, the third world is thus investing directly in the USA. Thus, when the USA 'invests' later in that country, say, by buying up the telephone system, it is, in effect, buying that country's assets with its own money. This is only mentioned in passing to show how Byzantine the whole thing is. It would even be hugely humorous if the health and welfare of so many people in the third world were not being sacrificed to keep the game going. Without attaching any purely political value judgement to it, this process must strike the reader as dreadfully inefficient. It should be possible to come up with a less costly system.

The need to establish an economic basis for human rights

Thus much of the inequity in health between the first world and the third world has come about through the system of debt from the first world to third-world nations. If we wish to make access to healthcare global, then, clearly, a more efficient system for the distribution of the benefits of production has to be found.

Various third-world countries have tried to buck the system, but since they have done so individually, they were – in most cases – easily isolated and picked off one by one by the first-world money lenders. Peru, for instance, got rid of its maverick President García – who tried to rule that debt repayments would not be allowed to exceed 10% of export earnings – and now Peru is hopelessly enmeshed in IMF debt. It had less money in 1993 to spend on schools and hospitals than it did in 1989 and yet a greater demand for those two facilities (George and Sabelli, 1994). This is because the debt repayments, which are not touching the principal borrowed, are so great. In Cuba, Fidel Castro never defaulted on Cuba's international debt, but wrote a book about the problem in 1982. It is even arguable that Cuba would have got away with simply not paying, for two reasons: its population was small, only about 10 million back then and it would have been easier for Citicorp Bank (the New York bank affected) to write the Cuban loan off as a bad debt than for the USA to become enmeshed in what would have been a protracted war so soon after the unpopular war in Vietnam had come to an end.

Suppose that a huge country like Brazil tried this approach. What would happen? The Brazilian debt produces interest payments that constitute about 23% of the profits of Citicorp (*Wall Street Journal*, 1991). Such a loss would seriously compromise the US domestic economy. Would the USA go to war? Who knows, but it hardly bears thinking about. It is difficult to see how anyone would benefit from doing so.

Consider also the case of Zimbabwe, which tried to take a tough line on the IMF. It managed to hold out alone for four or five years, but is now deeply in debt. Indeed, Zimbabwe's case illustrates yet another aspect of the sheer disadvantage of this way of running global finance: corruption. Financial institutions, even honest ones, cannot be expected to make rules and conditions relating to the ethical behaviour of their own governments or those of their debtor nations. Their professional concern has to be the correct legal protocols in the administration of the money. Since, in many third-world nations, the ruling élite is already sharply divided from the great mass of citizens, the temptation to indulge in corruption once the money comes in must be wellnigh overwhelming.

First the goods, then the people

We have seen that the third-world debt not only undermines the bases for healthy communities in the third world, but also in the first. The third world is forced into pushing its hard-won basic products onto a hostile world market, where the price is determined in competition with similar products from other equally indebted third-world nations. Because this leads to reduced return per unit of produce, the producers back in the third-world country are driven to even more desperate efforts to produce more – at immediate cost to their health, social integrity and environment, and at an ultimate cost to those aspects of life in the first world.

But, of course, there is a limit to how bad things have to get before people simply give up and flee their country. The limit, we know, is quite extreme. People do not usually flee their home and country, their sense of belonging, their language and culture, for fun. Young people may do so more readily, but they usually return to their own community once the adventure wears thin. However, the systematic stripping of living standards in a country will gradually force increasing numbers of more established people to flee for good. We are not talking here about political refugees, but about economic refugees. In the UK our treatment of – and social attitudes towards – asylum seekers often overlooks our own involvement in their original flight from home.

In real terms we might ask why this distinction is important. The British Home Office is greatly exercised about the difference to the extent that would-be refugees seeking asylum in the UK must prove that they did not flee their country only because they could no longer make ends meet there. This is especially ironic when it is reasonable to argue that one reason that the supplicant cannot make ends meet at home is because the first world has distorted his country's economy through IMF-imposed economic restructuring to pay back debt.

It is beyond question that there has been a substantial increase in migration of people from the third world to first-world countries since the end of World War II, and it is not unreasonable to attribute at least some of this to international debt. In a sense, we go into a country and take more and more of its goods until eventually, in desperation, its citizens start to follow the goods out.

The impact of emigration on a society's health

It is important to consider the effect on the home country of its citizens fleeing in large numbers. Although it is true that the very poorest feel the strongest immediate reason to leave, emigration costs money. There is therefore a tendency for a third-world society in this kind of predicament to become subdivided as follows. The most wealthy – usually those in government or closely linked to it – are generally doing very well. They would favour IMF and World Bank loans, firstly, because they probably benefit directly from them themselves and, secondly, because it strengthens their control at the top. A broad band of middle-level citizens have some money but are disadvantaged by the general economic situation. They have enough money to avoid total desperation, but are worried by the prospect of the fragile situation worsening and leaving them stranded. In addition, they are likely to have had secondary education at least and to face with some degree of confidence the fact that, if they do emigrate, they will have to learn English (or one of the other first-world languages) to seek employment.

But if large numbers of this middle-level group do take the opportunity to leave, their country is bereft of many of its former middle managers, teachers, healthcare personnel and so on. When the author was in Jamaica in 1987, on a United Nations Education, Scientific and Cultural Organization (UNESCO) contract, the only two children's clinics within a 20-mile radius of where he was living closed down within a week of one another. Both clinics had been progressively deteriorating for the previous five years because of cutbacks in health-care services instituted by a government striving to comply with IMF restructuring dictates. Similarly, their capacity to hire local cleaners had been reduced so much that basic hygiene was frequently ignored. However, the final closure occurred because all the staff emigrated to Canada. Not one of them was going to a job for which they had been professionally trained, but to do unskilled work for which they could earn much higher pay and guarantee that their children were able to attend school.

In such parlous situations, what tends to happen is that the absolutely poverty-stricken are driven to heroically desperate measures, such as crime (to secure money for a passage), stowing away and so forth. They leave because there is literally no alternative. On doing so, they often leave dependants behind. Usually, the intention is that, once the economic refugees have managed to lie their way into a first-world country and secure employment, they can start sending money to their families. In the meantime the latter live even more precariously than they did before the breadwinners left.

The people just above the level of desperate poverty, but still grindingly poor, observe that they had better hold on just a bit longer to see if they can avert disaster. In one third-world country after another this author has seen this sort of scenario unfold, and what it does to community empowerment and individual self-esteem hardly bears discussion. These last, of course, are two critical factors in sustaining physical and psychological health.

Wars, health and the debt

As Lalonde (1974) observed, in setting out the conditions which must prevail before health promotion can be effective, it is obvious that a society involved in military conflict cannot practise health promotion. Although it would be extremely difficult, if not impossible, to prove statistically that IMF restructuring programmes in the third world in the context of the international debt actually cause wars, a link can certainly be hypothesised.

Large parts of the world have been at war almost without break since World War II ended in 1945. Some of these wars have been between nations and of the 'classical' type, with identifiable armies, but most have been 'civil' wars and less 'formal'. Almost none of them have been regarded as being newsworthy, but their reality is nonetheless reflected in epidemiological data from the third world, for it is in the third world that most of these conflicts are taking place. There have been some newsworthy wars – Korea, Vietnam, the Gulf War, the Jewish Arab Wars and Iraq, for example – but the under-reported ones have been no less destructive for all that. One has only to consider the conflict between the Iraqis and the Kurds, or the Tutsis and the Hutus, to gain some idea of the magnitude of the problem.

It would be oversimplifying things outrageously to claim a simple set of reasons for these conflicts. For instance, conflict over resources is neither the only nor the most important factor of many of these events. But economic problems which induced mass migrations, starvation and wide-scale environmental damage will certainly exacerbate any other causes promoting conflict (Zwi and Ugilde, 1991). It is instructive to look at a list of the two dozen most highly indebted third-world nations and to note which ones were involved during 1990/1991 in warfare (*see* Table 2.3). The table also lists countries according to the debt service ratio (DSR) on the same basis. The DSR is calculated by working out the percentage of repayments or export earnings. The DSR gives a very clear idea of the disruption caused to the community life and values in a given country by the debt. The debt rankings are from 1989 data (World Bank, 1990).

Although structural readjustments generally serve to draw money away from health initiatives and thus prevent their development, it is also plain that by far the most expensive items on which borrowed capital is spent are armaments. This, accordingly, keeps the public sector (principally health and education) starved of funds. We therefore have a situation in which some consequences of debt repayments (such as environmental destruction, loss of domestic produce, emigration) exacerbate social tensions and thus create an 'enemy within' for the government of the debtor nation. But the debt is incurred (at least partly) in order to try to repress military insurgency. It is very much a chicken-and-egg scenario.

Furthermore, as long as third-world nations are faced with the problem of having to produce for exports in exchange for dollars, the arms trade will prove an irresistible attraction if the country concerned can produce the goods. In fact, it is almost as lucrative as the drugs trade and yet strictly legal. It is beyond the remit of our concern in this book to speculate how third-world nations gain the stocks of arms to sell, but a passing comment on it will serve to show how destructive it is of attempts to establish global peace – a precondition for equity in health. Some third-world nations accumulate huge arms supplies from wars fought in their territory. For years after the rout in Vietnam, Vietnamese arms dealers profited handsomely by selling discarded – but perfectly usable – war materials to other third-world countries for dollars.

When third-world countries import arms they do not always buy them from first-world countries, but they always pay in dollars. In terms of profits made by the first-world banks, therefore, this makes little difference. For instance, in 1990, India was the fourth most indebted nation in the world and yet it was then a leading (in terms of

Table 2.3: Debtors at war

Ranking of third-world states by gross debt	(US $ billion)	War, 1990–1991	Ranking of third-world states by DSR	%	War, 1990–1991
1 Brazil	(113)	–	1 Nicaragua	96	Yes
2 Mexico	(113)	–	2 Somalia	81	Yes
3 Argentina	(65)	–	3 Mozambique	72	Yes
4 India	(61)	Yes	4 Madagascar	64	–
5 Egypt	(54)	Yes	5 Guatemala	63	Yes
6 Indonesia	(54)	Yes	6 Algeria	62	–
7 China	(45)	Yes	7 Côte d'Ivoire	61	–
8 South Korea	(44)	Yes	8 Ghana	59	–
9 Turkey	(37)	Yes	9 Uganda	53	Yes
10 Nigeria	(32)	–	10 Mexico	53	–
11 Venezuela	(30)	–	11 Myanmar	52	Yes
12 Philippines	(28)	Yes	12 Niger	51	–
13 Algeria	(28)	–	13 Bolivia	46	Yes
14 Thailand	(25)	–	14 Congo	46	–
15 Israel	(24)	Yes	15 Brazil	44	–
16 Chile	(22)	Yes	16 Honduras	42	–
17 Peru	(21)	Yes	17 Jamaica	42	–
18 Morocco	(21)	Yes	18 Colombia	41	Yes
19 Malaysia	(20)	–	19 Uruguay	41	–
20 Pakistan	(18)	Yes	20 Argentina	40	–
21 Colombia	(17)	Yes	21 Indonesia	39	Yes
22 Iraq	(15)	Yes	22 Kenya	37	–
23 Côte d'Ivoire	(15)	–	23 Venezuela	37	–
24 Ecuador	(13)	–	24 Ethiopia	36	Yes
25 Vietnam	(12)	–	25 Philippines	35	Yes
26 Turkey	(35)	Yes	27 Nigeria	35	–

DSR = debt service ratio. Sources: OECD, 1990; World Bank, 1990

US dollars) arms importer (Wulf and Wulf, 1990). Of course, it has now gone one step better and has produced its own nuclear weapon – as has Pakistan. No doubt such developments have immensely enhanced healthcare among its own people and the prospect of health equity throughout the region!

Of course, we have not yet even considered the possibility that the debt itself may cause a cash-strapped third-world country to go to war. An apposite example of this is the first Gulf War. To support the war against Iran, Iraq borrowed extensively from other Arab states, including Kuwait. When that conflict had subsided, Kuwait tried to claim back its loan, to the tune of about US $12 billion. Now, Saddam Hussein had long wanted to annex Kuwait and – as was said at the time – if Kuwait had been noted as a producer of carrots rather than of oil, no doubt the first world would not have felt the 'moral' need to defend Kuwait when Iraq struck. Obviously, the debt was not Saddam's only motivation for going to war, but it was certainly a major factor.

Even if the reader considers the war in Vietnam a bit outdated, let us look at the more recent wars between third-world countries, but set in motion and/or exacerbated by their unequal financial involvement with the first world. I refer to such wars as are still running in the Democratic Republic of the Congo, the Côte d'Ivoire, Sierra Leone and the Solomon Islands – to say nothing of Iraq and of the Israeli–Palestine conflict. The Solomon Island conflict has been well described in economic terms by the World Bank, which reported on it in a rather upbeat manner in 2003. The reader is left to judge; the report is exactly as it appeared in the source cited:

> *The Solomon Islands have struggled with inter-ethnic tension since independence in 1978, although violent conflict only broke out in late 1998. About 20 000 people were forced to abandon their homes. In June 2000 there was a coup, and violence continued particularly in remote rural areas.*
>
> *The effects on the economy and the well-being of the people have been marked. Modest growth in national income has turned into severe decline. Net inflows of foreign direct investment declined from US $33.8 million in 1997 to US $1.4 million in 2000. By 2001, there was a net outflow of US $5.1 million. Debt grew by almost 50% between 2000 and 2001. While aid is about 23% of gross national income, the debt burden is about 58% (see Figure 2.1).*

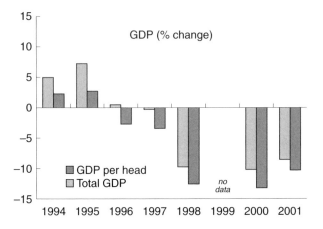

Figure 2.1:   The declining economy of the Solomon Islands at war. Source: Asian Development Bank, Asian Development Outlook. GDP = Gross domestic product

> *The Solomons are far behind on the Millennium Development Goals. Particularly in remote areas, declining funding of essential social services has adversely affected health and education indicators, now the lowest in the region. Maternal mortality rates are particularly high. New vulnerable groups are emerging such as those displaced by the conflict, the unemployed, especially women, and youth.*
>
> *More than two years later, Australia and a few other Pacific neighbours offered to send in a small peacekeeping force. The Solomon Islands parliament approved the force on July 17, 2003. By the end of 2003, a measure of stability had been restored. This may be the chance to prevent conflict as a driver from becoming conflict as a maintainer of chronic poverty. (Source: World Bank, 2003.)*

References

Asian Development Bank (2005) Solomon Islands data profile. *Chronic Poverty*. Institute for Development Policy and Management, University of Manchester, p. 45.

Bunyard P (1985) World climate and tropical forest destruction. *Ecologist.* **15:** 37–42.

Castro F (1982) *La Deuda Internacional es una Deuda Impagable* [*The International Debt is an Unpayable Debt*]. Government Publications, Havana.

Christian Aid (1998) *The Jubilee 2000 Petition*. Christian Aid, London.

GATS Watch (2005) GATS and the WTO Ministerial in Cancun in Sept. 2003. Available from Paulus Potterstreat 20, 1071 DA Amsterdam, Netherlands www.gatswatch.org. Accessed 2 September 2005.

George S (1992) *The Debt Boomerang*. Pluto Press, London.

George S and Sabelli F (1994) *Faith and Credit: the World Bank's secular empire*. Penguin, London.

Kissinger H (1999) US Financial Globalization – The Way Forward. Speech given at Trinity College, Dublin, as reported in the *Irish Times*, 14 October.

Lalonde M (1974) *A New Perspective on the Health of Canadians*. Information Canada, Ottawa.

Leggett J (ed.) (1990) *Global Warming: the Greenpeace Report*. Oxford University Press, Oxford.

Myers N (1989) *Deforestation Rates in Tropical Forests and their Climate Implications*. Friends of the Earth, London.

New York Times (2001) Drug trade supports terrorism. 24 May.

Organization for Economic Cooperation and Development (1990) *Financing the External Debt of Developing Countries: 1989 Survey*. OECD, Paris.

Organization for Economic Cooperation and Development (2000) Financing the external debt of developing countries. *Technical Notes*. 11: 75–88.

Rachman J and Bloch E (eds) (1974) *Multinational Corporations*. Trade and the Dollar Publishers, Chicago, IL.

Sanders D (2005) Primary Healthcare and Health Systems Development: strategies for revitalisation. Paper given at International People's Health University, 13 July 2005, Cuenca, Ecuador.

Shoup L and Mintel W (1977) Shaping a new world order. In: *Monthly Review Press*, Imperial Brains Trust, New York, NY.

United Nations Children's (Emergency) Fund (UNICEF) (1992) *Children for Health: children as communicators of the facts of life*. UNICEF, Geneva.

UNICEF (1998) *Communities for Development: human change for survival*. IB Taurus Press, New York, NY.

UNICEF (2000) *The State of the World's Children 2000*. UNICEF, Geneva.

UNICEF (2003) *The State of the World's Children 2003*. UNICEF, Geneva.

Wall Street Journal (1991) US vulnerable on foreign loans. 13 June.

World Bank (1990) *World Debt Tables for 1989–90*. World Bank, Washington DC.

World Bank (1990) *Debt Tables 1989–1990*. World Bank, Washington, DC.

World Bank (2003) Solomon Islands data profile. In: *Chronic Poverty 2004–2005*. Department of Economics and International Development, University of Bath. p. 47.

Wulf A and Wulf H (1990) The trade in major conventional weapons. In: *World Armaments and Disarmament (SIPRI Yearbook)*. Oxford University Press, Oxford.

Zwi A and Ugilde A (1991) Political violence in the Third World – a public health issue. *Health Policy and Planning*. 6: 203–317.

Chapter 3

The environment: our ultimate arbitrator

Environmental unsustainability

As stated in the Preface, we are, for the first time in our history, becoming acutely aware of a rather unpleasant referee, in the form of our degraded environment, standing at the sidelines shouting 'Time!' By that I mean that there are serious environmental constraints on our decision making with respect to the way we run the world. Most basic to this is global warming and the need to monitor more carefully what we do to the atmosphere.

As most school pupils now know, the ordinary processes of photosynthesis in green plants allow them to generate oxygen and accumulate sugar (glucose) by using up carbon dioxide and water in the atmosphere. The relevant equation is:

$$6CO_2 + 6H_2O + \text{sun energy} = C_6H_{12}O_6 + 6O_2$$

What this means is that six molecules of carbon dioxide from the atmosphere are combined (using energy from the sun) with six molecules of atmospheric water to produce one molecule of glucose (stored in the plant for its own growth and energy needs) and six molecules of oxygen are released as a by-product. In other words, photosynthesis enables green plants to use up carbon dioxide to produce and store sugars while releasing oxygen as a result. Herbivorous animals eating the plants thus gain sugar, which they break down by respiration into carbon dioxide and water vapour (breathed out), which provides them with energy (originally derived from the sun) and which originally held those molecules together as a sugar molecule. Carnivorous animals similarly get their energy from the sun, but more indirectly, by eating herbivores. Over billions of years this process produced our current ambient atmosphere, of which nearly 20% is oxygen.

But, as shown in Chapter 2, the current systems of trade globalisation are leading to the wholesale destruction of the earth's forest cover (thus radically decreasing the amount of carbon dioxide that is being recycled into oxygen), greatly increasing the carbon dioxide levels in the atmosphere. In fact, it is worse than that, because we are not only preventing carbon dioxide molecules from being used up by photosynthesis every time we cut down a tree, but we are adding extra carbon dioxide molecules by running the machinery that chops down the tree. Obviously, this is a no-win situation and cannot be sustained for long. So a major component of addressing the issue of inequity in trade and its negative impact on health in the third world is to address the environmental crisis that we have been busily creating.

This is a huge issue and almost all of our large-scale industrial processes, such as excessive use of internal combustion engines (for cars and trucks, but most especially for aircraft), will come under closer environmental scrutiny as more people become aware of the problems. In this chapter, a number of enormously unsustainable practices presently linked to globalisation are considered. Overuse of aircraft is one practice that is widely ignored, and today it is becoming routine for people to fly long distances on vacation or business. It is interesting to note that recent advances in computer technology render much of the latter unnecessary. Also, many people now dine on a huge array of exotic foods out of season because of our heavy reliance on air freight. Between 2000 and 2004. there was a 12-fold increase in air cargo miles flown. We shall now look at this aspect more closely.

The environmental cost of air transport

Siegle (2005), writing in the *Observer Magazine*, made the observation that, 'Thanks to low-cost airlines and super-size jets, the world has got smaller. Unfortunately, it has also got a lot hotter!' The reason that flying is now so cheap is that most governments (including the UK) do not charge tax on the high octane petroleum that commercial aircraft guzzle so prodigiously. Nor do airline passengers pay VAT on air tickets, nor do they pay tax on the duty-free goods sold at airports and even on some flights. It would not be incorrect to say that governments, including the UK, are thus complicit in this massively increasing assault on our environment. If the true cost of, say, a return flight from London to Edinburgh were calculated, factoring in fuel taxes, VAT and so on – never mind the more difficult-to-measure environmental costs (effects on asthma rates, noise pollution, for example) – the ticket price would not be widely affordable.

But governments are not likely to adopt such anti-business steps, and there would be a (heavily manipulated) public outcry if they did. It falls to the readers of books like this one to consider alternatives. In the short term, for instance, much greater use can be made of trains and ships for long-distance travel, and we could try and make more imaginative use of local farm produce. These matters will be discussed in Chapter 6.

But just how environmentally damaging is our modern love affair with air transport? Aviation is the fastest growing source of carbon dioxide emissions – currently about 5% of the EU total. It is estimated that by 2010, any progress that we have made through the Kyoto agreements will have been wiped out. It is worth noting that, in the UK, the government's stated objective is to cut carbon dioxide emissions by 20% by 2010. Air transport alone will scupper that target unless we take serious steps to curtail it. In his book *How We Can Save the Planet* Hillman (2005) comments rather laconically that a one-way flight from Paris to New York would use up about 25% of our legitimate (under the Kyoto agreement) annual carbon dioxide emissions quota. Fly back again and you have used up half. Even without air transport, however, the problem is immense.

It needs to be noted as well that carbon dioxide emissions are not the only thing producing global warming. We could mention methane, produced in small quantities by human flatulence, but in environmentally significant quantities by the same process, by both cattle and termites. The dramatically destructive levels of clearing huge tracts of Brazilian rainforest in order to raise beef cattle for McDonald's (and other hamburger chains) has significantly elevated methane emissions from cattle, to say nothing of carbon dioxide emissions caused by deforestation.

Can carbon dioxide emissions be traded?

There have been various attempts to balance the harmful emissions books by trading average emissions of greenhouse gases between countries. Although mathematically satisfying, it is difficult to see how this can really help. In the 1970s and 1980s, one solution put forward was that the USA, say, could balance out its extravagant production of carbon dioxide by 'owing' a calculated number of 'pollution points' to countries which produced less than agreed averages. But such procedures can only be transitory, and they create huge inequities in trading power and health. It is even more futile to argue that, within one country or territory (say, the EU) such an arrangement would make sense.

In the UK, latest figures show that the government is not making progress with such emission controls. It is even falling further behind. The *Financial Times* Stock Exchange (FTSE) top 100 companies account for 1.6% of the world total of carbon dioxide emission equivalents as of 2005. Only five of these firms, though, account for 70% of that total. The firms are, in descending order: Shell (UK), British Petroleum, Scottish Power, Corus and BHP Billiton (Houlder, 2004).

An attempt was made to organise some sort of trade-off strategy in 2005, which required the largest carbon dioxide emitters to begin trading as described above. The EU Emissions Trading Scheme was set up in January 2005, for carbon dioxide emissions. The UK government set a carbon dioxide emissions limit that was assigned to 1000 electricity generating companies and other heavy energy users. Each company has a fixed allowance and if its carbon dioxide emissions exceed that level it has to buy further allowances from other companies that are emitting less. In this way, a financial penalty is introduced for overproduction of carbon dioxide emissions, but this is only a paper trade-off. It does not actually reduce local emissions of carbon dioxide. As pointed out in an editorial in the *Morning Star* (2005), even this limited scheme actually leads to more carbon dioxide emissions. Companies that produce below their limit are simply selling their excess capacity to dirtier producers, establishing yet another market place in which a profit can be made out of pollution.

The effect of all this, of course, is that people's energy bills increase, the world becomes hotter, the weather becomes more extreme and thousands of people, especially in the third world where there are fewer health facilities, will die as a result. The same sort of profligate exploitation of environmental resources by the first world is evident with respect to water, as will be discussed below.

Water, water everywhere – but not to drink

The reader is no doubt aware that fresh water is not a commodity to be taken for granted worldwide. Very few humans have water on tap, and many of those who do have no guarantee of its potability and freedom from infection. In most of the places in which the author has been privileged to be of service, all except the very wealthy people have to carry water for long distances for domestic necessities. Diarrhoea, caused by infected water, kills large numbers of infants and frail old people. These deaths – and the inconsolable suffering attendant on them – are largely preventable, but not under the present inbuilt inequities between the wealthy and the poor nations.

Even in countries such as the Dominican Republic, a major tourist spot for wealthy people from the first world, tap water is often unsafe. The wealthy buy safe water in large bottles, regularly delivered to hotels and to their homes, but the great bulk of the population routinely experience typhoid and other water-borne diseases. Death by such causes is common – yet within hailing distance of thoughtless pleasure-seekers, who know nothing about it. The ostentatious displays of wealth in that country have to be seen to be believed. While working over there in medicine during 1985–1987, I constantly met tourists and the local wealthy expatriate community, who resolutely did not want to know what was happening so close at hand. They were 'enjoying themselves' and found such information 'unsettling'. They would return to the USA and the UK and elsewhere, and rave about how lovely the Dominican Republic was. The degraded lives of the dispossessed had nothing to do with them. In a fair world, of course, such attitudes can have no place. Let us take a brief historical look at the development of our relationship with the planet's water supply.

Growing first-world control over water

Before the European industrial revolution of the eighteenth and nineteenth centuries, people all over the world had a somewhat similar association with water. They relied almost exclusively on water available at, or near, the surface of the earth. Rivers, lakes and springs constituted the most commonly used sources. Indeed, it was widely assumed that these sources were inexhaustible, due to the evaporation–rain cycle. However, in Europe and North America, rapid industrialisation quickly changed all that. Large quantities of the easily accessible water were needed to run generators and other machinery. River sources – and, more recently, ocean coastlines – became polluted and unfit for use. Sewerage systems became necessary as larger concentrations of people grew up around ports and factories. In the first world, we began our long-term exploitation of underground water resources (aquifers*) and even the elaboration of huge desalination enterprises.

As Craig (2002) points out, the first world and some of the third world are now exploiting aquifers at a prodigious rate. Without some kind of international mediation and control, it is difficult to see how this can continue. Aquifers contain about 97% of the planet's water supply. Increasingly, these very sources face the danger of pollution, but simply their rate of use must cause alarm. Water tables are now dropping at the rate of three metres annually, according to some estimates. In the prairie states of the USA, and the prairie provinces of Canada, up to 15 metres of water are being extracted yearly, while the natural replacement rate of 1 cm per year is only 1/1500 of that.

It is anticipated that aquifer sources of water in the USA and Australia will be exhausted by about 2030. Of course, the impact of this depletion will not be felt first or most adversely in the first world, but in the nations of the third world. As Craig (2002) points out, Beijing's water table has dropped 59 metres in only 40 years. Of 2.6 million wells in the province of Beijing, and in two neighbouring provinces, more than 100 000 wells had run dry by 2000. Even more obscenely, the use on an industrial scale of this non-renewable source strictly for profit in the first world is increasing year by year. It has to be curbed, and soon. Even some first-world people are now imminently threatened by it – but, of course, it is the poor who bear the greatest brunt of this exploitation.

How about a game of golf?

Golf course maintenance requires extraordinary quantities of fresh water, and some lavish clubs built in poorer countries for the use of wealthy tourists threaten local people as far apart as Fiji, North, South and Central Africa, Jamaica and the Philippines. The matter has recently become serious even in some first-world countries. In the past two years, the USA, Canada and the UK have expressed concerns about it. Giles Trimlett (2004), a reporter from the *Guardian* newspaper, commented on the situation in the Mediterranean resorts:

> *These places attract millions of tourists set on improving their golf.*
> *Each of an estimated 200 golf courses situated around the southern*

---

* Aquifers refer to water-bearing rocks, or rock complexes, underground.

Mediterranean consumes the same amount of fresh water as a town of 1200 people, according to a report released on 7 July 2004, by the World Wide Fund for Nature (WWF). In the southeast of Spain – already an arid region – it is planned to build 89 more golf courses. Greece is planning 40 more and Cyprus eight. Responsible individuals and agencies are seriously calling on people not to patronise such establishments. The report's author, Lucia de Stefano (2004), describes the region as wilting under the pressure of 135 million tourists to beaches stretching from northern Morocco and Spain to Greece, Turkey, Cyprus and Tunisia. It is further anticipated that this figure will at least double by 2024.

'The tourist industry depends on water, but it is at the moment destroying the very resource it needs,' asserted Holger Schmidt, a WWF spokesman. He also pointed out that the vast expanse of land being taken out of use by being concreted over for leisure centres is adding greatly to the level of ecological damage. It is understood that the exploitation of the entire coastline for the tourist trade will push urban boundaries further inland, displacing subsistence farmers and destroying the few remaining coastal wetlands and lagoons. Another EU study, reports the same article, states that over 50% of the wetlands (vital for waterfowl breeding and conservation) of France, Greece, Italy and Spain have already disappeared.

In the poor countries of North Africa, steps are already underway to imitate the tourism of the northern Mediterranean. Water demand increase over the next 20 years will have such an impact that even underground (aquifer) water supplies may well be exhausted by about the year 2050. Morocco's Moulouya Estuary currently embraces about 400 hectares of marshlands, but looks likely to be destroyed in the rush for dollars from the first world's tourists. Threatened with extinction will be the monk seal and such rare birds as the slender-billed curlew and Andalusian hemipode.

At present, tourism accounts for 7% of all pollution in the Mediterranean Sea. Already this has caused major upsurges in ear, nose and throat infections among endogenous people of the area concerned. Hepatitis and dysentery are also on the increase. The negative ecological impact is now rapidly accelerating. Building is proceeding at levels that are not ecologically sustainable. For instance, Tunisia is planning to double the 85 km already built-over for tourists and hence remove this land from food production.

France has built 335 000 second homes – largely for big spenders from the other first-world nations – in only 20 years. Spain is said to be building 180 000 homes a year – 40% of them for UK residents. In 27 towns along the Alicante coast in Spain, a stable domestic population of 150 000 is pushed up to 1.1 million (almost seven-fold) every August. Water consumption in the Balearic Islands has increased to 35 times the 1980 levels (de Stefano, 2004).

What about climate change?

In the *Guardian* (2001) we read that the melting of the polar ice-caps, attributed to global warming, is now proceeding at such a rate that some of our largest cities (such as London and New York) face imminent inundation. Some third-world countries (Bangladesh, for example) have been suffering this effect for years, caused largely by carbon dioxide emissions from the industrialised first world, and this has barely made the news. But now we are seeing that the way we live our lives in the first world is directly threatening its own citizens.

Obviously, many of our largest and most advanced cities were built in, or near, sea-coasts for access to ports for trading. But, as Sir David King, the government's chief global warming scientist said in an article in the *London Evening Standard* (King, 2004), carbon dioxide emissions are now causing an accelerating diminution of the polar ice-caps. Within only a matter of 20 years or so, the water levels around London could rise by five to ten metres. A rise of three metres would be enough to wipe London off the map. New York is similarly threatened.

Sir David went on to say that, in 2004, there was enough carbon dioxide in the atmosphere to melt both ice-caps. Of course, melting is a comparatively slow process, which accounts for the predicted time-gap. He commented, 'Climate change is the biggest problem that human civilisation has faced for 5000 years. When the Greenland ice-cap goes, the sea levels will rise six to seven metres, but when Antarctica melts, it will rise another 100 metres.'

Sir David King made these comments just after returning, as the UK government's chief adviser, from Moscow, where he had been trying to persuade the Russian government to ratify the Kyoto Agreement to fight climate change. The reader is no doubt aware that the USA was the first major carbon dioxide producer to refuse to ratify it. As will be discussed later in this chapter, such abstentions render the Kyoto Agreement almost useless. Suffice to say, it underlines the point (*see* Chapter 6) that any effective solution must be internationally mediated to be effective. We cannot be held to ransom by the short-term political and economic interests of individual nations or their corporations.

Sir David King went on to point out that recent scientific studies have confirmed the worst predictions about global warming. Records from the three kilometre-deep Antarctic snow core show that, during 'ice ages', the carbon dioxide in the atmosphere remained almost static – at about 200 parts per million (ppm), which rose to about 270 ppm during very warm periods. But human intervention, especially with the onset of industrialisation, has pushed carbon dioxide levels so high that they have effectively broken the cycle. In the 1990s, carbon dioxide levels reached 360 ppm, and they are now at 379 ppm. They are increasing at a rate of three ppm a year. That means that they are now at levels not experienced on earth for 55 million years – when there was no ice at all on the planet.

The consequences of lack of global control

We do not need to look far to see how national economic interests currently create environmental problems for us all. US President George W Bush was 'elected' on an incomplete ballot-count in 2000. His campaign was very much supported by his country's oil interests, which had felt restricted by some of the attitudes of the previous Democrat administration, for instance the latter's favourable disposition towards the Kyoto Agreement.

One of President Bush's first actions on taking office was to withdraw US pledges to reduce carbon dioxide emissions, calling it a 'mistake' (Brown, 2001). He also abrogated legislation intended to control sulphur dioxide emissions from US petroleum refineries. Sulphur dioxide not only produces acid rain when it combines with atmospheric water but, within a short radius around the plants concerned, has a deleterious impact on the health of residents. Who, one might ask, would be living that close to something as unattractive as a petroleum refinery? It would largely be people far down the economic ladder in the USA – black people, Mexican migrants (legal and illegal) and so on. George W Bush finally got that legislation passed at the height of the panic and outrage over the two terrorist attacks on the World Trade Center, widely referred to as '9/11' due to the American system for recording dates. In that horror, more than 3000 lives were lost – many of them nameless illegal migrants who cannot even be traced – while the legislation cutting limits on sulphur dioxide emissions may well have killed many more than that number of American poor in the first year of its enactment. Without some sort of worldwide control over such issues, we are surely doomed. Consider, for example, the Bhopal disaster in India, from which many thousands still suffer ruined lives and health, to say nothing of the multitudes who died in the event itself. Bhopal is the capital city of Madhya Pradesh state in central India. In December 1984, Bhopal was the site of the worst industrial accident in history, when about 45 tons of the dangerous gas methyl isocyanate escaped from an insecticide plant in Bhopal that was owned by the Indian subsidiary of the US firm Union Carbide Corporation. The gas drifted over the densely populated neighbourhoods around the plant, killing many of their inhabitants immediately and creating a panic as tens of thousands of others attempted to flee the city. The final death toll was estimated at as high as 2500 lives, and local medical facilities were overwhelmed by about 50 000 other people who were disabled by respiratory problems and eye irritation resulting from exposure to the toxic gas. Investigations later established that substandard operating and safety procedures at the understaffed plant had led to the catastrophe (Wilson and Roberts, 2001).

Needless to say, that plant, which was producing insecticides for the profit of US interests and was selling most of its insecticide to customers in the first world, was situated in a third-world country for sound business reasons. In the USA there are labour laws protecting workers and a reasonably vigorous trade union system to see that they are applied. However, in the third world, and especially in the poorest nations, such legislation either does not exist or is not enforced if it is going to interfere with trade. Health and safety provisions, which are accepted as required in a first-world society, are often regarded as dispensable luxuries elsewhere.

Under impartial global control, in which the welfare of people is a dominant criterion, such exploitation would be far less likely to occur. For instance, governments or other agencies within a given economic interest cannot even be allowed to be the sole arbiters of what happens to the natural resources of their own country. Not long after President Bush (Junior) came to power, considerable discussion arose – and is still being considered – about the possibility of extracting oil from huge reserves recently discovered in Alaska. This would be a godsend for American oil corporations and probably a great relief to the fuel-hungry American people generally. At present, great uncertainty attends continued US access to oil from overseas and especially from the Middle East. As the OPEC nations did in the 1970s, the overseas oil producers are in a position to hold the USA (the world's greatest user of oil, by far) to ransom. What could be better for the USA than to have the security of an increase in its own supply?

But, extracting oil from Alaska would probably destroy, or seriously compromise, the National Park there. Many species unique to the area would face the possibility of extinction. The local rivers and wetlands, as well as coastal fishing interests, would face pollution on a large scale. The use of that much extra oil would greatly exacerbate global warming. Siberia faces the same problem. In both places – and in a number of similar regions – the permafrost is weakening quickly under the impact of global warming and this is now undermining the foundations of buildings and of huge stretches of highways. Bridges and other large structures, such as railway lines, are threatened, as are port facilities. In the Rocky Mountains region in both the USA and Canada, thawing is resulting in massively destructive rock falls, mudslides and even the collapse of whole mountainsides (Craig, 2002). Much of the approach to global warming used here by this author has been informed by Craig's brilliant little book. Although only 52 pages long, it is a pocket-sized gem of effective exposition and argument.

These events often result in the formation of temporary dams, which either divert water flow – jeopardising housing and/or agriculture – or form huge lakes, which can suddenly break free of the blockage, wiping out communities in massive deluges. The impact of such 'flash floods' on electrification, water supplies, railways, roads and telephone communications is already common in some parts of Central America, where governments have often sacrificed conservation policies and health and safety for international trade. Much of the latter, indeed, has stemmed from the need to repay IMF loans (*see* Chapter 2).

Financial consequences

Many third-world countries are hard put to recover from the effects of such disasters because of the vast costs of reconstruction they entail. It has been estimated by Godrej (2001) that such reconstruction costs will, by 2050, supersede the value of the entire world economy at that time. Insurance payouts alone stemming from climate-related claims have been doubling every decade since the 1960s. In 1964 they stood at $30 billion, due to 16 major disasters, but in 1991 the figure stood at $250 billion, as a result of 70 major disasters. These sums leave out the many secondary costs – many of them not even financially measurable. The Red Cross forecasts that indirect and secondary impacts of disasters like these may well be twice the cost of the direct losses (Godrej, 2001). In fact, climate-related insurance payouts, as opposed to claims, are anticipated to increase from today's $30 billion per year to $300 billion by 2050 (Dlugolecki, 2002).

Big tidal waves and tsunamis

These two phenomena are often confused and, since both are important to the concerns of this book, the author will discriminate between them. A *tsunami* is caused by an eruption (generally volcanic) on the ocean floor. If it is big enough, it can create one or several large waves, which then travel outwards along the floor of the sea. A *tidal wave*, on the other hand, is a rapid rise of sea level above predicted tidal levels, when water piles up with great force against a coast by powerful offshore winds. 'Storm surge' is regarded as a more correct expression than 'tidal wave'.

The *Guardian* (2001) carried an article on tsunamis, as cited by Craig (2002). There are, it points out, many notoriously unstable land masses on the planet, but one of the most noteworthy is the Canary Islands, which bears ample evidence of previous tremendous earthquakes. Cumbre Vieja is the name of their major volcano, and it is regarded by earth scientists as exceptionally dangerous. In one of its eruptions in 1949, a huge fissure opened in its west flank. At some future date it is expected that the resulting enormous and unstable mass of rock – twice the volume of the Isle of Man – will break free and slide into the sea, triggering the largest underwater wave ever recorded.

It is also considered inevitable by scientists that this will generate further giant waves moving westward, still under the surface. Once they have passed at high speed through the depths of the Atlantic, the waves will strike the shallows of the eastern seaboard of North America. By then, these waves will be several thousand kilometres in length and up to 50 metres high. One does not have to have a particularly profound imagination to realise what such a phenomenon could entail. Waves of that size and force would certainly wipe out life and settlement for several kilometres inland. They would not only affect the USA and Canada, but many other areas as well. Maybe all we are waiting for is the eruption of Cumbre Vieja, or a nuclear war.

Less dramatically, the rock could fall because of much more mundane human activities, such as human-induced torrential rains penetrating and weakening the fault line already exposed on the west flank of the volcano. Rock and mudslides like this are now not uncommon. Consider the collapse of the Las Casitas volcano in Nicaragua after a week of torrential rain, resulting from Hurricane Mitch in 1999. In that case, approximately 1400 people were killed but, fortunately, no storm surge took place – only because the mountain concerned was not on the coast.

In the USA in particular, there tends to be a cavalier attitude towards the issues raised at the Kyoto talks. Survey after survey carried out by US pollsters shows that, overwhelmingly, Americans would not consider giving up their unnecessarily large, petrol-guzzling cars. Their entire lifestyle is strongly consumer-driven, with the average American gobbling up non-renewable fuels and minerals at a rate of up to 80 times that of the average European, and much more than the average person from the third world. Indeed, as Craig (2002) so ably points out, 'unless greenhouse gases are reduced significantly, today's decision makers in the first world risk being guilty of inflicting on their own populations possibly the most appalling and sudden holocaust in human history'.

How much time do we have left for remedial action to have any chance of being successful? This is not easy to calculate. Even some of the less pessimistic earth scientists assert that, by 2050, about 75% of the world's people could be at serious risk, unless we act now.

The following two chapters will further illustrate the link between health, trade and human rights by considering two issues that affect both the first and the third worlds and thus allow the health impact discrepancies to speak for themselves. Thus, Chapter 4 is concerned with how first-world multi-nationals, often with IMF support, exploit mothers in the third world through the promotion and sale of breast milk substitutes, with melancholy results. This will be contrasted with the strenuous promotion of breastfeeding in first-world contexts as being the superior alternative healthwise. Chapter 5 reflects on the global pandemic of HIV/AIDS and offers a differential analysis of its impact in the first and third worlds.

References

Brown L (2001) *Bio-economy*. Earthscan, London.

Craig N (2002) *World Rescue – Climate Facts/Demand for Action*. Housmans Bookshop Publications, London.

Dlugolecki G (2002) Climate change and the financial services industry. Available at www.solstice.crest.org/renewables/gasifications-list-archive/msg03619.html. Accessed 10 July 2005.

Financial Times (2005) UK exceeding CO2 emissions limit. 29 July.

Guardian (2001) Gaynor T. Under the volcano. G2 section. 29 August.

Godrej D (2001) *No-nonsense Climate Change*. Verso Press, London.

Hillman M (2005) *How We Can Save the Planet*. Penguin, London.

Houlder V (2004) *Financial Times*. 23 November.

King D (2004) as quoted in: London 'among first to go' as sea level rises. *London Evening Standard*. 18 July.

Morning Star (2005) A really dirty deal (Editorial). 3 August.

Siegle L (2005) Plane speaking. *Observer Magazine*. 29 May.

de Stefano L (2004) *The Coming Water Crisis*. Pamphlet issued by the Worldwide Fund for Nature, Godalming.

Trimlett G (2004) Save the planet – don't play golf. *Guardian*. 16 July.

Wilson D and Roberts S (2001) *Five Holocausts*. Wellington, New Zealand.

Chapter 4

Mothers, milk and money

Powdered milk: a threat to third-world babies

The negative impact that powdered milk substitutes for babies can have on their health is now widely appreciated in the first world. Until about 1980, in many first-world countries, there had been a steady decline in breastfeeding as more and more mothers opted for bottle feeding. The arguments for it seemed persuasive – it allowed partners to share in the chore, especially at night, mothers could return to work or other activities during the day, it allowed mothers to maintain a better bosom shape and so forth. However, the weight of medical and scientific evidence began to move in the other direction as research established that breast-fed babies bonded better with their mothers and that breast milk carried certain immunological protections and nutritional values which powdered milk could not. Breastfeeding was also shown to be of great psychological and physiological benefit to the mother and allowed her endocrine balance to be restored better after the birth. For the past 20 years or so, the situation has begun to change, with an increase in breastfeeding in the first world.

While bottle feeding had been gaining ascendancy in the first world, it was virtually unknown in the third world, where breastfeeding had been routine from time immemorial. But, as popular educated opinion in the developed nations began to move away from bottle feeding, the powdered milk firms began energetically to establish a market for their products overseas. By the early 1980s there was considerable evidence of this. While working in Accra for UNESCO in the 1980s, the author noticed large, well-produced hoardings advertising a well-known milk powder for the bottle feeding of babies. The advertisements featured pictures of two mothers – on the left, a Ghanaian mother holding her baby to her breast, and on the right, another Ghanaian mother holding her baby in one arm while she bottle-fed it. The mother on the left was poorly dressed, had huge pendulous breasts and was decidedly down-at-heel and haggard. The mother on the right had small, tight breasts under a suit of clean and fashionable clothing, and appeared young, fit and very much 'with it'. Along the bottom of the hoarding was a strip reading: 'Which mother do YOU want to be?' The message, of course, was clear. What perhaps was not so easy to appreciate is that similar campaigns had run in the first-world nations during the 1940s and 1950s, but they had become less persuasive for several reasons. Among these were increasing access to education for Western women, a more discerning purchasing power among mothers and 'breast is best' campaigns. Non-governmental organisations proliferated in countries such as the USA and the UK* to provide tips to new mothers who had decided to breastfeed, and – above all – certain manufacturers of 'baby milk formulae' were being slated for trying to profit from people's ignorance. Life was becoming tougher for milk substitute manufacturers in the first world. They responded in two ways: by diversifying into production of commodities such as breakfast cereals and by shifting the milk powder business into the third world, where access to basic education for women was less available, and where nervous, recently formed indigenous governments were less likely to interfere.

Support for third-world services

Ghana was not the only (nor the first) third-world country to undergo this experience. Ministers of health and individual hospital directors in such countries found themselves being offered funding to establish maternity care units and even money to staff them, provided that the emphasis was to be on encouraging new mothers to bottle-feed. The whole package was made even more attractive with a programme under which mothers were given three weeks' free supply of formula when they left the hospital. Such an offer would be extraordinarily difficult for a cash-strapped third-world government to resist.

When the mothers returned home with their babies, however, certain problems arose. Many mothers, unable to afford further supplies of powder, would try to make the free supply last as long as possible. Generally this was done in one or both of two ways: they would make the formula for each feed more dilute than specified in the directions on the packet; or they would add other powders – such as corn meal or maize – to the commercial powder.

---

* In the UK, the Breastfeeding Help Line (01624 670383) gives direct practical assistance to parents having problems with breastfeeding.

This author often witnessed these practices and had a difficult time persuading some mothers that colour and texture of a powder were not sufficiently precise criteria by which to decide whether or not it could be used as a 'stretcher'. But yet more problems quickly made themselves felt at the village level.

Market forces, structural adjustment policies and private enterprise

Whilst in the maternity unit, the young mother would have usually been able to rely on the water supply she was using to mix the baby milk formula. But in the village a reliable source of clean water was much more problematic. Routinely, young babies died of enteric infections and diarrhoeas caused by use of polluted water. This risk greatly increased once mothers either added inappropriate stretchers to the formula or diluted it beyond the specified levels.

Moreover, as part of the World Bank structural adjustment policies, third-world client governments were encouraged to cut back on public sector spending and to push money into support for private initiatives. The cutbacks on public sector spending certainly knocked back large-scale rural water reticulation and purification plans. This is something that the author frequently witnessed first-hand throughout the 1980s, in a range of third-world countries.

But the return to the village of mothers who now needed a dependable supply of commercial milk formulae opened up new opportunities for rural private enterprise initiatives – something which IMF or World Bank loans were dedicated to encouraging. In Ghana, Kenya and Papua New Guinea – widely separated cultures with widely divergent ethnologies – the similarity of private-sector intervention in this context was astounding. After she has been back from maternity care for, say, two or three weeks, the new mother is likely to be running out of her free supply of formula. Of course, she cannot replenish her supply locally and must rely on a 'trader'. The 'trader' is a man (usually) who owns a pick-up truck, often kept in precarious running order by a combination of ingenuity, hay-binding wire and faith. Every fortnight or so, he will drive to the capital (or some other larger town) to purchase commodities ordered by people from the village and not available locally.

In short, he is an entrepreneur. His charges for each item so purchased must be enough to cover expenses – of which petrol is an obvious one – but will exceed that level by an amount dictated by 'market forces'. These are largely determined by how great the customer's need for the product in question is. In the case of young mothers, when their supplies of formula milk have dried up, their need is quite clearly a life or death one, as far as the baby is concerned. The author witnessed a mother being told that a package of Lactogen, costing one shilling and six pence in town, 30 miles away, would have involved her paying the trader four shillings. The negotiations were fearful to behold. The trader even offered the mother five shillings for the baby, confident that he could sell it at a profit in town. The author intervened, handed over what currency he had – enough for 11 packages of Lactogen at the going rate – and then had to leave. He often wonders what happened when that supply of Lactogen ran out, but was assigned to another country only a day or so later. Let us now consider the matter in more analytic terms.

The status of breastfeeding in the third world

Obviously, the desire to lead a healthy life is a worldwide phenomenon, along with the wish to raise well-nourished children and provide them with opportunities for the future. Most governments regard it as a priority to invest in public health measures and programmes to improve health. However, resources are usually scarce while so many other demands are made upon them.

It is a truism that breastfeeding is a natural resource that can have a major impact upon health and family planning goals. If more women were to breastfeed their infants for longer periods of time, fewer infants would die, women and children would be healthier and public health and family planning programmes would save money (Labbock and Nazro, 1995).

Generally speaking, there has been an increase in many countries of women opting for the breastfeeding route. This has come about largely because national policy makers, health professionals, support groups and families have begun to recognise the many benefits of breastfeeding, and have strengthened their support for it. Over and above those global trends, though, a north–south divide is evident. There are far more industrialised countries in which breastfeeding rates are low but rising, and third-world countries in which breastfeeding rates are high but falling. If considered globally, the figures reflect a decline in rates of breastfeeding.

We now address the benefits of breastfeeding and outline the main causes of the decline in global breastfeeding rates, identifying specific actions that health workers and policy makers can take in order to promote and preserve this natural resource.

Breastfeeding as part of the health promotion agenda

It has been stated (Jones, 1997) that breastfeeding is one of the purest forms of health promotion and is of vital importance to infants and their mothers for nutritional, immunological and psychological reasons (Cunningham, 1987). Breast milk is unique in its composition, varying its contents during and from one feed to another according to an individual baby's needs. These compositional changes are set in motion by the mother's hormonal response to her own infant's needs and also to the climate of the country, altering the proportion of fluid in relation to the local temperature and humidity. In situations in which an infant feeds directly from the mother's breast, the milk cannot easily be contaminated whatever the quality or quantity of a local water supply. It is also true that breast-fed babies are protected against diabetes, pneumonia, ear infection, polio and many other conditions.

From the mother's own point of view, the message is also supportive, for the practice has an immediate positive effect on maternal health, reducing post-partum haemorrhage. In addition, it is generally believed to reduce the risk of pre-menopausal breast cancer (Newcombe *et al.*, 1994), osteoporosis (Cumming *et al.*, 1985) and some forms of ovarian cancer (Schneider, 1997).

Additionally, we know that exclusive breastfeeding during the first six months usually results in hormonal suppression of ovulation, and this prevents pregnancy before the mother's menstrual cycle resumes. With longer intervals between births, mothers and babies are healthier, resulting in lower maternal and infant mortality, and lower fertility rates. This confers greater maternal control in spacing births, giving mothers more time to regain their strength and health status. It also allows them to give appropriate time and energy to older children whilst sustaining breastfeeding for the youngest one. A frequently quoted statistic is that infants born less than two years after their next sibling are twice as likely to die as infants born after this gap. A three-year gap increases this protection (Rustein, 1984).

Third-world economics and breastfeeding

From the purely management perspective, there are important economic advantages in breastfeeding to families, health providers, family planning programmes and national budgets. Consider also the cost of substitutes: where one-half to one-third of the population live in poverty in large urban areas, the cost of manufactured breast milk replacements to provide adequate nutrition, plus the necessary feeding equipment, constitutes a significant portion of a family's income. Other members of the family may be inadequately fed as a consequence of buying infant formula, or conversely, the infant formula may be watered down to make it go further, with obvious malnourishment consequences. The death rate is higher, malnutrition starts earlier and the morbidity incidence is greater in formula-fed babies (Labbock and Nazro, 1995).

UNICEF (1997) states that if the 51% of Indian mothers who breastfeed exclusively were to stop doing so, replacing all the breast milk with infant formula, it would cost US $2.3 million. In Indonesia, a study in the 1980s calculated that the mothers produced over one billion litres of breast milk annually; equivalent supplies of commercial milk would cost US $400 million. The loss of savings in health costs and reduced fertility rates related to breastfeeding were estimated to cost another US $120 million. In Haiti, where just 3% of infants are breast-fed, infant formula costs US $10 per week per child – more than twice a typical income.

A UNICEF (1998) study has been carried out which shows cost comparisons in improving the maternal diet by an additional 500 calories per day above the mother's normal diet so that she can breastfeed properly, versus the equivalent cost of formula for the baby. In India it was found that five days' worth of extra food cost less than 15 rupees (45 cents), whereas the comparative cost of infant formula over the five days was 130 rupees (US $3.70). In the Philippines, the Jose Fabello Hospital saved 8% of its annual budget (US $100 000) within one year of taking steps to promote and support exclusive breastfeeding.

It was stated by the Director-General of the WHO, in 1985, that the lives of 1.5 million infants could be saved every year if, for the first six months of life, infants were breast-fed exclusively and given no solids or other liquids, not even water. To ensure continuing health development and survival after six months of age, it is preferable that breastfeeding continues, supplemented by nutritious food (Jong-Wook, 2004).

Impact on the third world

Trade and exploration, of course, generated the spread of European values, including incorrect health education messages. By the end of the Victorian era, this situation had become almost worldwide. Jones (1997) states that in Malaysia, in 1926, British nurses reported that 'some mothers had not even seen a clock and those who had could not understand what it had to with the feeding of an infant'. Needless to say, the cost of infant formulae has national financial implications as well as for families. Expenses devoted by developing countries to the import of infant formula often use up scarce foreign exchange needed for other essential priorities. Furthermore, it costs the country more in the use of scarce healthcare funds because they are treating illnesses relating directly to the decline in breastfeeding.

Current statistics suggest that approximately 44% of infants in the developing world (fewer in industrial countries) are exclusively breast-fed. Among the factors responsible for the decrease in breastfeeding rates worldwide, surely the relentless promotion of breast milk substitutes by 32 multi-national infant feeding companies, such as Nestlé, Abbott-Ross, Mead Johnson, Nutricia and Wyeth, must be the greatest. We know that in a few developing countries in which breastfeeding rates remain high, such as Rwanda (90%) and Burundi (89%), there is little marketing of powdered milk (*see* Table 4.1).

It was not until the 1970s and 1980s that the negative effects of infant formulae on infant health and survival rates first became apparent. Along with this came the identification of the fact that advertising had a role in the promotion and use of infant formula, especially in developing countries. In 1977, frustration in response to aggressive global marketing led to a consumer boycott specifically against Nestlé, and this spread from the USA to 10 other countries, including the UK. Eventually, this action led to a reduction of inappropriate advertising and promotion of baby milk substitutes. These developments have been central in the fight to protect and promote breastfeeding.

Table 4.1: Breastfeeding rates in developing countries*

10%		>50%	
Developing countries with exclusive breastfeeding rates of 10%	(%)	Developing countries with exclusive breastfeeding rates of >50%	(%)
Niger	(1)	Rwanda	(90)
Nigeria	(2)	Burundi	(89)
Angola	(3)	Ethiopia	(74)
Côte d'Ivoire	(3)	Tanzania	(73)
Haiti	(3)	Uganda	(70)
Central African Republic	(4)	Egypt	(68)
Thailand	(4)	Eritrea	(65)
Cameroon	(7)	China	(64)
Paraguay	(7)	Mauritania	(60)
Maldives	(8)	Bangladesh	(54)
Senegal	(9)	Turkmenistan	(54)
Dominican Republic	(10)	Bolivia	(53)
Togo	(10)	Iran	(53)
Trinidad/Tobago	(10)	India	(51)
Guatemala	(50)		

Data refer to infants under four months of age.
Source: UNICEF, 1997

The WHO response

The WHO approved the *International Code of Marketing of Breast-Milk Substitutes* in 1981. The document was drafted by the WHO together with UNICEF. Non-governmental organisations and representatives of the infant food manufacturers had contributed as well. In theory, the *Code* established minimum standards to regulate marketing standards by setting out the responsibility of companies, health workers, governments and others. It also provided standards for the labelling of breast milk substitutes. The most salient provisions of the *Code* were:

- no advertising of breast milk substitutes
- no free supplies of samples
- no promotion of products through healthcare facilities
- no contact between company marketing personnel and mothers
- no gifts or personal samples to health workers
- no words or pictures idealising artificial feeding, including pictures of infants on labels of the products
- information to health workers should be scientific and factual only
- all information on artificial feeding, including labels, should explain the benefits of breastfeeding and the cost and hazards of artificial feeding
- unsuitable products should not be promoted for babies.

New mothers are particularly vulnerable to psychological and commercial activities, and providing free or subsidised supplies of infant formula, bottles and teats on maternity wards must have eroded the confidence and good intentions of many mothers to breastfeed. Clearly, for the minority of children who cannot be breast-fed, say, because the mother is infected with HIV/AIDS, infant formula is an important product. However, sales and promotional activities relating to infant formulae have sometimes been based on false claims as to their value in comparison to that of breast milk. It is of no small interest that, included in the provisions of the *Code*, is the statement that health facilities must never be involved in the promotion of breast milk substitutes and that free samples should never be given to pregnant women or new mothers.

An important guardian of the *Code*, and of compliance with it, is the International Baby Food Action Network (IBFAN), set up in 1998. Every three years IBFAN publishes a report on levels of compliance with the *Code*. One of the acknowledged deficiencies of the *Code* is that it is weak in certain areas, and the first-world milk substitute manufacturers have not been slow to exploit these loopholes while ostensibly complying with the it. Their one dominant theme over this period was the emphasis on fatty acids found naturally in breast milk, but imitated (derived from fungi, algae or fish oil) and added to the formula, purportedly to make babies more intelligent! This mixture, given the trade name FORMULAID, was produced by Martek and supplied to almost all the main milk substitute producers. Eleven of the 16 international companies discussed in the IBFAN (2004a) report jumped on the bandwagon of selling 'intelligence in a bottle'. All are cashing in on the emotional desires of parents to have bright children.

Martek, the main supplier of these oils and additives to most such breast milk substitutes, actually stated the following in 2002 (IBFAN, 2004a):

> *Infant formula is currently a commodity market with all products being almost identical and marketers competing intensely to differentiate their products. Even if FORMULAID has NO benefit, we think it would be widely incorporated into baby milk formulae as a marketing tool and to allow companies to promote their product as 'closest to human milk'.*

After Martek had written this in 2002, its sales rose by 183% in only nine months. It took independent researchers two further years to establish that the additives have no definite health benefits.

A long-term aim was that the *Code* would gradually be enshrined in legislation. But its progress in being translated from minimum voluntary provisions into national law has been desperately slow. In September 1997, only 17 countries globally had approved laws which put them into full compliance with the *Code*. In 1997 came a report entitled, 'Cracking the *Code*', published by the Interagency Group on Breastfeeding Monitoring (IGBM). This highlighted violations of the *Code* and work still to be done. IGBM is made up of 27 organisations, including churches, health experts, academic institutions, agencies such as UNICEF UK, Save the Children Fund, Voluntary Service Overseas (VSO) and others. 'Cracking the *Code*' is the first major community-based study undertaken of the prevalence of *Code* violations and of the urgent need for enforcement. Serious violations of the *Code* by multi-national infant food manufacturers in four countries – Bangladesh, Poland, South Africa and Thailand – are thoroughly documented. By implication, this publication also highlighted the negative impact of World Bank promotion of structural adjustment policies.

Breastfeeding versus market forces

Featured in the IGBM report was a statistical analysis of interviews with 800 pregnant women and new mothers, and also with 120 health workers in 40 facilities in each country. Many violations of the

Code emerge in their accounts. For instance, infant formula companies had been distributing marketing literature promoting formula over breast milk and giving free formula to maternity hospitals and mothers at ratios of one in 12 mothers in Poland and one in four mothers in Thailand. Giving free samples of milk substitutes to new mothers represents a particularly insidious way of promoting formula, because even a few days of feeding infant formula using a teat and bottle makes a baby fussy about taking the breast. The mother's lactation will naturally have become reduced through lack of stimulation and may not be capable of increasing again. In this way the mother is then forced to feed and buy formula when the free supplies cease, at great cost to the baby, the family and the state in both health and economic terms (IBFAN, 2004b).

The whole sordid process is facilitated if the free samples are actually given to the mother by paramedical staff at a clinic or hospital. Obviously, health workers such as doctors and nurses are seen as giving the product the health professionals' stamp of approval by handing out these 'gifts' but in doing so they are acting unethically by condoning the violation of the *Code*. Unsurprisingly, the International Association of Infant Food Manufacturers (IFM) soon complained that the IGBM report was biased and unscientific. The reader can easily ascertain, however, that the experimental design and the random sampling framework used to investigate the violations were standard epidemiologically sound techniques of the kind used by governments and research organisations, the WHO, UNICEF and others for assessing the prevalence of health conditions internationally (IBFAN, 2004a).

Reacting to modern research showing falling breastfeeding rates, the global strategy of UNICEF's Baby Friendly Hospital Initiative (BFHI) was launched with 'The Ten Steps to Successful Breastfeeding' (Gockay *et al.*, 1997). Established in response to resistance to change, implementation has nevertheless been slow, especially in industrialised countries. Getting health professionals to change their ways can be far more difficult than getting mothers to acknowledge the benefits of breastfeeding. However, it has been unambiguously established that infant formula manufacturers have used their marketing practices to exploit medical mistakes, such as the unnecessary administration of dextrose or formula.

Implementation of the BFHI in Chile has raised breastfeeding rates of 4% in 1985 to 25% one year after its launch in 1991. A national survey in 1996 suggested exclusive breastfeeding rates of 40% for the first six months after birth. Training health workers became a crucial part of the equation, as was strong support from the Ministry of Health and sustained advocacy from UNICEF, and the introduction of the BFHI is gradually spreading globally with the developing countries showing the way forwards (UNICEF/WHO, 1989).

We are now in a stronger position to consider the cost, in both health and economic terms, and to make an analysis of some of the insidious reasons for the decline in breastfeeding. As we have seen, the decline in breastfeeding began in the 'civilised world' and has gradually spread to the developing countries, but only after having been promoted as the best start for babies because of the extent that mothers from wealthier countries were represented as rearing their babies on infant formula. Unquestionably, the *Code* has had the effect of making health professionals aware of insidious promotion of baby milks. Seductive presents of pens, calendars, obstetric calculators and posters, all bearing the name of infant formula companies, will have appeared to many mothers to be an endorsement by health professionals of the wisdom of using formulae.

It has been in third-world countries that the awareness of the major damage caused by the drop in breastfeeding rates was first seen. Similarly, it is in third-world nations, in which the state of health and economy are more fragile, that the remedies are now commencing. The response to the BFHI and legislation relating to the *Code* have been implemented far more effectively in those countries than in their industrialised counterparts.

Breastfeeding worldwide

Mothers, as a group, have been disempowered over the centuries, and as advocacy needs to start 'from the bottom up', help with the practicalities of teaching breastfeeding is vital to facilitate a restoration of this empowerment. One approach would be the promotion of a more holistic approach to childbirth and infant feeding, with the latter being seen as a natural process requiring only minimal interference. Of course, such matters need to be approached sensitively, and in full awareness of cultural and other contextual factors.

Research has shown that few reasons why women do not breastfeed are nominated, and they fall mostly into three categories:

• women who cannot do so for medical reasons, such as breast cancer or AIDS

- women who resolve not to breastfeed because of personal or socially induced resistance
- women who cannot survive the initial difficulties which sometimes arise in early days, despite wishing to breastfeed.

No one doubts that there will always be some role for the use of infant formulae, but there is considerable divergence in the views of health professionals about the amount of information given, regarding formulae and the sterilisation of feeding equipment, antenatally. For instance, the *Code of Conduct – Guidelines for Professional Practice*, published in 1996 by the United Kingdom Central Council of Nursing, Midwives and Health Visitors (UKCC), states: 'the registered practitioner must not practise in a way which assumes that only they know what is best for the patient, as this can only create dependence and interfere with an individual's right to choose'. In other words, a politically correct awareness of the autonomy of patients compels nurses to respect whatever choices patients make. Gough (1996) claims that overemphasis on an individual basis to promote breastfeeding could be seen as victim blaming, if not unethical, of a nurse. Susan Bates (1996) of the Health Visitors' Association stated:

> Patients are entitled to choose how to feed their infants and as much information as possible should be provided to help parents make informed choices. Having made their choice, mothers should be given as much help as possible to establish infant feeding with minimum difficulty – it must not become a witch-hunt.

Undoubtedly, the huge multi-national infant formula companies have a major influence on feeding practices worldwide and also have the vast resources to promote them. On the other hand, the financial resources for promoting breastfeeding tend to be minimal and mostly generated by voluntary bodies, such as IBFAN. Possibly, legislation is the key, and if the codes of practice for manufacturers can be monitored more closely and more countries bring in enabling legislation, matters will improve more quickly. Money hitherto spent on counteracting multi-national advertising can be utilised in more appropriate ways. One obvious such initiative could be providing the kind of practical support to initiate breastfeeding from which new mothers now benefit in first-world nations.

With no obvious legal restraints preventing it, the instant formula manufacturers' lobby continues wilfully to misinterpret the *Code*. Despite the word *International* in its title, the manufacturers' body insists that the *Code* applies only to third-world countries. These companies still continue to promote breast milk substitutes unethically and to flout the *Code*: whilst this continues, concerned parties are likely to maintain pressure, perhaps by maintaining the boycott of Nestlé, which produces 40% of the world's baby milks.

The two-pronged attack needs to continue, both 'bottom up' and 'top down'. The bottom up approach involves the local communities, empowering women to make informed choices about the infant feeding and also to give them back the skills that were once second nature with the aid of practical tuition and support. The top down strategy is the global action of organisations and pressure groups continuing to monitor and publicise violations by baby milk manufacturers, and to continue boycotts of the same. However, a cautionary note is necessary here. Firms do respond to popular pressure, as their profit margins depend on goodwill. When faced with boycotts, many companies diversify into other areas of less questionable production. To boycott these products also is thoughtlessly counterproductive. In a sense, the companies should be rewarded for such a stategy. In the 1990s Nestlé, for instance, shifted into the breakfast cereal market and took over the manufacture of Shredded Wheat, formerly a NABISCO (National Biscuit Company) product. In 1997 that breakfast cereal was the only one that had nothing but good said about it on health grounds (Cannon, 1988).

Now third-world countries are taking the lead over industrialised countries in implementing changes that will raise breastfeeding rates. All things considered, this should not be so surprising, as the effects of the possible damage caused by infant formula feeding are more catastrophic in these countries. It might be appropriate to finish with a comment from the Right Reverend Simon Barrington-Ward, until recently Chair of the International and Development Affairs Committee of the Church of England's General Synod:

> *For babies everywhere, the benefits of breastfeeding are undisputed. But for babies in developing nations breastfeeding is imperative: their very survival depends on the immune boosting properties of mother's milk. For them, infant formula is not just inferior; it can cause disease or even death. Poor families often over-dilute costly formula with unclean water and mix it in unclean bottles, adding to the risk. Yet despite international pleas and a marketing code agreed in 1981, manufacturers still market infant formula with other substitutes unethically around the world. It is time for them to stop. (Comments made in a sermon at Evening Prayer in Southwark Cathedral, 16 May 1991)*

There has been no really sustained improvement and the rest of this chapter deals with one of the worst offenders, Nestlé. There are others, but Nestlé controls 40% (as of 2004) of the market globally.

Nestlé and its impact on the third world

As we have seen, breastfeeding has everything to recommend it. It is cheap, involves no transport costs and is the least polluted feed available. Breast milk also carries protection against many infections to which babies would otherwise be prone. Because it provides optimal nutrition, it can reduce the entire family's poverty – which is a major cause of malnutrition. It has been shown to reduce the risk of breast cancer (Boral, 2002). In fact, both UNICEF and the WHO estimate (2004) that 1.5 million lives can be saved annually through increased breastfeeding (IBFAN, 2004c).

But, breast milk has to compete in a rapidly growing market for breast milk substitutes, now worth US $10.9 billion (Gaudrin, 2001). The *International Code of Marketing of Breast Milk Substitutes* (WHO, 1981) and its resolutions, and other policies which attempt to protect breastfeeding and ensure responsible marketing of breast milk substitutes, challenge such growth and are opposed by companies. Nestlé controls approximately 40% of the baby food market, and, as the world's largest food company (with over 11 000 brands of processed foods), is able to exert a powerful influence on government policies and market trends. For more than two decades Nestlé has been dogged by criticism of its baby food marketing and is the target of an international boycott campaign. Because of this Nestlé has curbed some of its more blatant malpractices, removing pictures of babies on infant formula tins and stopping some media advertising. It has also spent millions of dollars on public relations strategies which include sponsorship, glossy brochures and attempts to link its name with and to influence the UN system. Nestlé's sustainability review, its infant feeding in the developing world and its infant feeding policy are all examples which present Nestlé as a responsible company, even a leader in sustainable development and environmental protection – a company that is eager to listen to criticism and to act on it. But all these documents fail to stand up to scrutiny. In reality there has been no real change of policy nor any commitment to a marketing strategy that will match the public relations promises.

Worldwide independent monitoring consistently shows that Nestlé, more than any other company, systematically violates the *Code* and its resolutions, promoting its products in many ways which damage infant health. The few limited changes Nestlé has made do not counterbalance the harm caused by its marketing and its persistent undermining of legislation and trading standards which seek to protect infant health.

The author is grateful to IBFAN for permission to use the following material, which was published in 2004.

> *Despite Nestlé's persistent reference to its compliance with the International Code, the company's policy and instructions, against which all staff behaviour are measured, are substantially weaker than the International Code and the subsequent relevant World Health Assembly Resolutions. During a public hearing at the European Parliament in November 2000 UNICEF's Legal Officer stressed how much more stringent the International Code is in approach, coverage and scope than Nestlé's policy and instructions. Nestlé boycotted the hearing. The following ten points show the questionable intentions of Nestlé's whole approach.*
>
> *1 The International Code applies to all nations, not just developing countries. Nestlé's policy and instructions apply only to what it calls 'developing countries' and so do not cover countries such as Poland, Hungary, Korea or Taiwan. For the smallest, most defenceless of consumers, such double standards make no sense at all.*
>
> *2 The International Code covers all breast milk substitutes, including any products marketed in ways which undermine exclusive and sustained breastfeeding. Nestlé's policy and instructions apply only to 'infant formula'.*
>
> *3 Nestlé's policy and instructions fail to include the ten Resolutions which have been passed at the World Health Assembly since 1981 and have the same status as the International Code itself. They are important because they clarify, update and strengthen the International Code's provisions in the light of research and current marketing practices. WHO has confirmed that the International Code and the Resolutions enjoy equal status and should be read together as one and the same document.*
>
> *4 Nestlé ignores the fact that the International Code was adopted as a minimum requirement to be implemented in its entirety. Where countries have laws stronger than the International Code, companies must abide by those stronger laws. However, where countries have weaker measures Article 11.3 of the International Code requires*

companies to ensure that their conduct at every level conforms to it, and to do so independently of any measures taken by governments.
5 Hundreds of violations of the International Code from 14 countries were published in IBFAN's report, Breaking the Rules 2001, and were brought to Nestlé CEO, Peter Brabeck's personal attention in 2001. He has dismissed the vast majority as invalid and, so far, done very little to end the practices which endanger infant health.
6 Nestlé claims to be the first company to implement the Code. However, it is the responsibility of governments to implement it and then the companies must comply with it. Nestlé, more than any other company, undermines government efforts to implement the Code and Resolutions. In India, for example, it not only lobbied against the law for many years, but when facing criminal charges over the language and text of its labelling, it issued a Writ Petition against the Indian government, attempting to have key sections of the law struck down, including some articles directly implementing the Code. The Writ Petition still stands and some see it as an attempt to delay the legal action taken against Nestlé which could see its Managing Director imprisoned. In Zimbabwe, before the government brought in its strong law in 1998, Nestlé threatened to pull out all investment, arguing that 'it would not be economically viable for the company to continue operating under such regulations'.
7 Nestlé's policy and instructions refer only to direct consumer advertising of infant formula. The International Code calls for a ban of all promotion of all breast milk substitutes – either direct to mothers, to health workers or to the public. The aim is to protect health and ensure that parents receive independent, objective information about infant feeding. Under the International Code, health workers are responsible for advising parents on infant feeding.
8 The International Code calls for all information about and on products to be restricted to scientific and factual matters with no idealising pictures or text, such as 'maternalised' or 'humanised'. One advertisement for Nativa infant formula, intended for health workers in Côte d'Ivoire, claimed that Nativa is even better than breast milk: 'Nestlé: Meeting the need for certain micronutrients which the human organism cannot produce, but which are needed to orchestrate a gamut of physiological functions essential for optimal development'. Mr Brabeck dismissed the violation.
9 Nestlé's Sustainability Review states: 'Free infant formula donated over the past 12 months was only for social welfare cases'. As long ago as 1994, World Health Association (WHA) Resolution 47.5 stated

that there should be 'no donations of free or subsidised supplies of breast milk substitutes ... in any part of the healthcare system'. Breaking the Rules 2001 found free or low cost supplies of infant formula in ten of the 14 countries studied. On 1 May 2002 UNICEF staff found boxes and boxes of donated Nestlé's Bear Brand Prebio 2 follow-on formula in a Bangkok hospital. None of the staff seemed to be sure why the samples were donated, but the excuse was given that they might be for mothers infected with HIV. Less than 3% of mothers are known to be infected with HIV in Thailand. The mothers who are infected are provided with free formula which is purchased through the Ministry of Public Health in a bidding process and made available to all hospitals. There is therefore no need for hospitals to accept free supplies from companies.

10 All over the world baby food companies aggressively promote expensive, packaged 'complementary foods' resulting in mothers using them as breast milk substitutes, often feeding them through a bottle. In 1994 WHA Resolution 47.5 stated that complementary feeding should be fostered from six months of age, and in 2001 WHA Resolution 54.2 emphasised the importance of exclusive breast-feeding for six months and the use of indigenous nutrient-rich foodstuffs. At its AGM in April 2001, Nestlé promised to encourage exclusive breastfeeding for six months, but has since stepped up its promotion of Cerelac complementary food from four months in many countries. Full colour glossy advertisements, with idealising pictures and text and offers of free samples, appear regularly in Indian newspapers with blatant health claims about micronutrients. In 2001 and 2002 the Codex Alimentarius draft guidelines (Codex sets global food standards) proposed that health claims should not be used on labels of foods for infants and young children. The 2002 WHA Resolution (55.25) specified that the marketing of micro-nutrients should not undermine breastfeeding or optimal comple-mentary feeding. (IBFAN, 2004c)

Nestlé's use of the HIV/AIDS pandemic

Some businesses will exploit absolutely calamitous situations to their own advantage and – except for the fact that Nestlé controls such a huge percentage of the market – it is probably no worse than many other firms in its cynical use of the desperation and fear caused by HIV/AIDS in some of the poorest countries.

Nestlé has been using the HIV/AIDS pandemic to push the use of its infant formula, Pelargon, in Africa. It launched a Nutrition Institute in August 2001 and has been visiting policy makers in southern Africa, making unsubstantiated claims that Pelargon's high acidity will kill germs and that this makes it safe to use with infected water. Nestlé has done much to distort mothers', health workers' and policy makers' perceptions, playing up the risk of HIV infection from breastfeeding and playing down the risks of artificial feeding. IBFAN believes that, when partnerships are formed between non-governmental organisations and companies such as Nestlé, which have a vested interest in mothers choosing artificial feeding in the context of HIV, women's rights to truly independent and objective information on this subject are undermined. The WHA Resolution passed in May 2001 (WHA 54.2) reaffirmed this right, stressing the need for independent research into HIV and stating that mothers should be protected from commercial influences. In 1999, Stephen Lang, Deputy Director of UNICEF, commented:

> *Those who make claims about infant formula that intentionally undermine women's confidence in breastfeeding are not to be regarded as clever entrepreneurs just doing their job, but as human rights violators of the worst kind.*

Other questionable practices revealed by IBFAN

We have already considered the problems that an unreliable and impure supply of accessible water poses for third-world mothers using powdered milk. This author has often, in his third-world country work, found that only people who can pay for individual lots of bottled water have access to reasonably reliable water. But what happens when firms like Nestlé also corner this market?

Nestlé is the world's largest manufacturer of bottled water, with over 50 brands and 16% of a fast-growing US $33.7 billion market. Nestlé faces criticism about its damage to the environment and local ecosystems in many countries. The promotion of bottled water can undermine commitment to the provision of affordable piped water. Irresponsible promotion and labelling and brand names such as 'Pure Life' can falsely imply sterility, undermining breastfeeding and safety messages about boiling water for babies. Bottled water is not sterile and must be boiled before use. Mineral water is unprocessed and may have unsuitable levels of salts for use in infant feeding.

At its AGM in March 2002, Nestlé faced criticism from shareholders about the impact of its water business on the environment and concerns from Perrier workers about the use of plastic bottles (supplied by Coca-Cola). Nestlé responded with promises to sell three to five million bottles of Perrier in China. In Brazil Nestlé has been accused of 'pillaging' the 'circuito das Aguas' (a Brazilian geological marvel) and 'destroying an eco-system which took nature thousands of years to create' (IBFAN, 2004c). Naturally, Nestlé is ever-anxious to counter such negative commentary by claiming that it is developing internal safety watchdogs.

According to the Nestlé sustainability review, Nestlé is instituting an ombudsman system. This could be a sign that it is recognising that it has a problem. However, this will mean nothing unless the terms of reference are clear. An internal ombudsman – paid by the company – is totally different from an independent ombudsman paid by a government or other party. The allegations of malpractice reaching up to senior management, provided by former Nestlé Pakistan employee Syed Aamir Raza, remain unanswered. Mr Raza claims he was threatened by Nestlé in 1997 when he challenged the company to stop its malpractice. He resigned soon after witnessing the death of an infant as a result of unsafe bottle feeding. Unless the ombudsman system is accompanied by a complete change of policy on Nestlé's part, employees will continue to be placed under intense pressure to maximise sales, as Mr Raza was. To protect someone like Mr Raza, an ombudsman would need to have greater power than the CEO Mr Brabeck, who is now the driving force behind the company. Mr Brabeck continues to make unsubstantiated attacks on Mr Raza's character.

Nestlé has refused to provide information about audits it refers to in the sustainability review, and readers must accept on trust that only four problems were uncovered. EME, the auditors called in to investigate in Pakistan in 2000, were specifically instructed not to look at the evidence of Syed Aamir Raza and were limited to interviewing doctors from a list provided by Nestlé. Baby Milk Action's offer to provide documentary evidence of malpractice, including the bribing of doctors, was not passed on to the auditors by Nestlé.

In IBFAN (2004b), the following comment appears:

> In July 2001 Nestlé and all the baby food companies cited as violating the International Code in IBFAN's report, Breaking the Rules 2001, were excluded from the FTSE4 Good Index for socially responsible investment.

All of these matters are more fully dealt with – and embrace companies other than Nestlé – in the IBFAN publication, *Breaking the Rules – Stretching the Rules* (IBFAN, 2004b). It presents evidence of violations of the *International Code of Marketing of Breast Milk Substitutes* (WHO, 1981).

References

Bates S (1996) Culture change. *Nursing Standard*. **10**: 17.
Boral V (2002) Breast cancer and breastfeeding: collaboration reanalysis of individual data. *The Lancet*. **July 360**: 187–95.
Cannon G (1988) *The Politics of Food*. Century Publishers, London.
Cumming SR, Kelsey JL and Nevitt MC (1985) Epidemiology of osteoporosis and osteoporotic fractures. *Epidemiology Review*. **7**: 178–208.
Cunningham A (1987) Breastfeeding and health. *Journal of Paediatrics*. **110**: 658.
Gaudrin B (2001) The booming market in breastfood substitutes. *Euromonitor*. May: 4.
Gockay G, Uzel N, Kayatark F and Neyzi O (1997) Ten steps for successful breastfeeding. Assessment of hospital performance, its determinants and planning for improvement. *Child: Care, Health and Development*. **23**: 187–200.
Gough P (1996) Heavy handed. *Nursing Standard*. **10**: 17.
International Baby Food Action Network (IBFAN) (2004a) Breaking the rules: stretching the rules. How does DHA-ARA get into formula? In: *Evidence of Violations of the* International Code of Marketing Breast Food Substitutes. IBFAN, Penang, Malaysia. Penang. Malaysia.
International Baby Food Action Network (2004b) Breaking the rules: stretching the rules. In: *Evidence of Violations of the* International Code of Marketing Breast Food Substitutes. IBFAN, Penang, Malaysia.
International Baby Food Action Network (2004c) Nice design – shame about the text: Nestlé's infant feeding policy and sustainability review – another PR cover-up. In: *Evidence of Violations of the International Code of Marketing Breast Food Substitutes*. IBFAN, Penang, Malaysia.
Jones E (1997) Cracking the Code – monitoring the *International Code of Marketing of Breast Milk Substitutes*. *Modern Midwife*. **7**: 27–9.
Jong-Wook L (2004) Published in International Baby Food Action Network (2004) *Breaking the Rules: stretching the rules*. IBFAN, Penang, Malaysia.
Labbock M and Nazro J (1995) *Breastfeeding: protection of a natural resource*. Georgetown University, Institute for Reproductive Studies, Washington DC.
Newcombe I, Allen G and Pearson L (1994) Lactation and a reduced risk of premenopausal cancer. *New England Journal of Medicine*. **330**: 81–7.

Rustein S (1984) Infant and child mortality: level, trends and demographic differentials. *WFS Comparative Studies No. 43.* 212–16.

Schneider AP (1997) Risk factors for ovarian cancer. *New England Journal of Medicine.* **317**: 558–9.

United Kingdom Central Council of Nursing, Midwives and Health Visitors (1996) *Code of Conduct – Guidelines for Professional Practice.* UKCC, London.

United Nations Children's (Emergency) Fund (1997) *Progress of Nations* www.unicef.org/pon97. Accessed 5 September 2002.

UNICEF (1999) *Statistical Profile of HIV/AIDS.* UNICEF, Geneva.

UNICEF (1998) *The State of the World's Children – Breastfeeding Breakthroughs – Tackling Malnutrition in Bangladesh – Protecting, Promoting and Supporting Breastfeeding.* UNICEF, Geneva.

UNICEF/WHO (1989) *Protecting, Promoting and Supporting Breastfeeding: The special role of the maternity services. (A joint statement).* UNICEF/WHO, Geneva.

World Health Organization (1981) *International Code of Marketing of Breast Milk Substitutes.* WHO, Geneva.

Chapter 5

The third-world face of HIV/AIDS

Capitalism: scourge of the third world

For a person in a first-world country to be diagnosed as HIV positive is a staggering blow. It would affect all their future relationships, family life and career prospects, to say nothing of their physical and psychological health and financial status. But, in most cases, such a person could still plan for the future and continue with many of their former activities. All of that, of course, is attributed to the availability of medical treatment, especially ARVs, and counselling. The picture, however, is completely different for most third-world people so afflicted. Indeed, the impact of HIV/AIDS in the first and third worlds is so different that they could almost be regarded as different diseases. A study of Table 5.1 reflects the wide differences in occurrence between the first world, where the figures are described in thousands, and the third world, where we are dealing with millions. The data is as of August 2004 (Lovich, 2004).

Table 5.1: Worldwide incidence of HIV/AIDS

Location	Numbers affected
Sub-Saharan Africa	26 820 000
South and south-east Asia	6.4 million
Latin America	1.6 million
East Asia and the Pacific	1.0 million
Eastern Europe and Central Asia	1.5 million
North America	995 000
Western Europe	600 000
North Africa and the Middle East	600 000
Caribbean	470 000
Australia and New Zealand	15 000
Total	40 million

Source: Lovich, 2004

We can see immediately that Africa alone accounts for nearly 75% of the cases. Only 20 or so years ago, HIV/AIDS was hardly heard of, whereas today it has already rolled back modest successes achieved by the third world in healthcare and is undermining the social fabric of thousands of communities, and even exceeds war as a threat to the lives of millions of children. It is estimated that in Africa another parent dies of HIV/AIDS every 11 seconds. Figures like that are almost impossible to comprehend. What it means is that orphans are being produced at industrial output levels (*see* Table 5.2).

Table 5.2:   Children orphaned by AIDS

Location	Numbers affected
Africa	11.0 million
Asia	1.8 million
Latin America and Caribbean	578 000
Total	13.4 million

Source: Lovich, 2004

During the night of 5 August 2005, BBC Radio 4 (the World Service) reported that six million people (mainly in the third world) require ARVs, but that only 300 000 receive them (only 5%). In South Africa in 1988, it was estimated that three in every 1000 pregnant women were HIV positive, a scandalous statistic in itself. But, by 2005, the figure was three in every 10 (BBC World Service, 2005).

At the 2004 International HIV/AIDS Conference in Bangkok, Kofi Annan warned that, without immediate international action, Asia will soon see rates of infection rivalling and surpassing those of Africa. Table 5.2 (Lovich, 2004) illustrates the trans-generational impact of this largely preventable scourge – a scourge maintained and enhanced by the globalisation of trade under the aegis of capitalism.

Africa's relationship with HIV/AIDS

As we have seen, collectively, the African nations have the highest incidence of the pandemic, but this obscures the fact that in that continent some communities are making heroic progress against it. I refer in particular to Uganda, but it is significant that Uganda was being heavily impeded by the WTO in 2004 when trying to provide its citizens with generic copies of ARVs produced and sold by first-world pharmaceutical companies at 22 times the cost. The US delegate to the WTO fought for eight months to stall negotiations designed to assess the safety and efficacy of much cheaper generic copies of the first world's anti-retroviral agents. As Flick (2003) reported:

> A long awaited trade deal to give poor nations access to cheap lifesaving drugs for diseases such as AIDS, malaria and tuberculosis was agreed on August 30th 2003, after eight months of stalling mainly due to US objections.

At that meeting of the WTO there were only 146 nations represented, and they all hailed it as a 'major breakthrough'. But some aid organisations were less enthralled. For instance, Médecins Sans Frontières argued that 'it threw up new legal, economic and political obstacles' to poor countries wishing to import (from other larger third-world countries, such as Brazil or India) cheap generic copies of patented drugs. In that respect, of course, it may still have been good news to US and other first-world pharmaceutical companies. Under the WTO, 'compulsory' licence patents for life-saving drugs cannot be waived for countries which could produce their own generic copies. It is also illegal to import or export them. The agreement came about in the face of a joint statement from African nations, which pointed out that 2.2 million Africans had already died from AIDS between the Doha meeting, where the matter was first raised, in 2001 and 2003. What are we in the first world doing about it? An indication is given in the Chronic Poverty Report (2004–05) (*see* Box 5.1).

Box 5.1   Are rich countries and their citizens really committed to reducing poverty? Targeting MDG 8

The bold Millennium Declaration from 189 countries that 'We are committed to making the Right to Development a reality for everyone and to freeing the entire human race from want' is not yet matched by bold actions on the part of the developed world.

Goal 8 of the Millennium Development Goals declares the establishment of a global partnership for development. It promises the Least Developed Countries (where the greatest concentrations of chronically poor people live) tariff and quota-free

continued

access for their exports; an enhanced programme of debt relief for HIPC and cancellation of official bilateral debt; and more aid for countries committed to poverty reduction.

What has followed this declaration? Trade talks at Cancun have failed as OECD countries refused to open up their highly protected agricultural markets; debt reduction has proceeded at a snail's pace; and rich countries have made promises of more ODA at Monterrey but have not committed anything like the necessary resources.

MDG Goals 1–7 – all of which are the primary responsibility of developing countries – have agreed targets that are regularly monitored. There is less emphasis on quantifiable targets, however, for MDG Goal 8, which is about what rich countries do.

MDG = Millennium development goals; ODA = overseas development assistance; HIPC = heavily indebted poor countries.

Some non-African third-world settings

Before dealing with the situation in Africa in greater detail, consider the situation in India, China and even the Russian Federation. The latter is of particular interest because, before the collapse of the Soviet Union, Russia had one of the finest statistics on health in the world. It now ranks at third-world levels. Within 10 years of the break-up of the USSR, the average life-span in that country had already dropped 12 years.

As Kofi Annan predicted, HIV/AIDS has made great headway in India and China. From 2000 until 2004, the AIDS pandemic advanced rapidly. The same thing is already happening in the Russian Federation. The latter has suffered a disastrous increase in poverty and an almost total withdrawal of its once excellent state-run health service since the collapse of the Soviet Union barely 15 years ago. This almost certainly is responsible for the rapidity of advance of AIDS in that country.

Altogether in India, China and the Russian Federation, AIDS rates are now increasing. Indeed, this is now having a severe effect on the not-at-risk group. Because of its uneven prevalence over all, infection is often easier than not. The Chronic Poverty Report (2004–05) asserts that low overall prevalence rates serve to mask huge local differences.

It is to be hoped that the Asian states (as well as the first world) learn from Africa's successes and failures. Yet again, this is an opportunity for the first world to make a more concerted, and less profit-driven, effort to ameliorate the situation. It is a global problem. We cannot stand aside from it. The UN programme for HIV/AIDS (UNAIDS) has stated that unambiguously (UNAIDS, 2003).

China presently has about one million people with HIV/AIDS. UNAIDS expects the incidence of HIV to soar in the context of ever-widening socio-economic disparities and massive amounts of migration. These prevalence rates are estimated to rise 10-fold by the end of the decade. In 2001, China launched a five-year AIDS action plan, signalling a growing recognition of the huge task at hand.

After South Africa, India has the most people living with HIV/AIDS of any country, an estimated 3.97 million as of the end of 2001, and rising. If HIV/AIDS is not brought under control, it is likely to undermine progress made in reducing poverty, particularly in the southern states. In July 2003, a National Parliamentary convention on HIV/AIDS was convened, in which over 1000 political leaders from mayors to ministers took part. The Executive Director of UNAIDS described the event as 'historic' (Chronic Poverty Report, 2004–2005):

> *Never before, in any nation of the world, has there been such a large and committed gathering of the leaders from every level of decision-making, dedicated to the common cause of fighting AIDS.*

Africa revisited

Despite the phenomenal successes of countries such as Uganda (MacDonald, 2005) over recent years, HIV is spreading exponentially in other areas of that continent. Over large regions, such as Sudan, Darfur and Republic of the Congo, viciously destructive wars are still being fought. This obviously undermines all of the involved communities first economically and then, because of that, healthwise. War has never been known as a particularly good context for human rights or gentlemanly behaviour and is an excellent breeding ground for HIV infection. It does not always require a war, though. Take Malawi as a case in point. The Chronic Poverty Report (2004–2005, p. 43) provides the following information:

> *The food crisis in Malawi in early 2002 resulted in several hundred, perhaps several thousand, hunger-related deaths. Starving Malawians*

resorted to eating unripe and unconventional foods, including flour fortified by maize cobs and sawdust, much of which made them ill. Malnutrition was high, not only among young children, older people and the ill, but also among working adults. An estimated 30% of the population required emergency aid.

The famine can be explained in two ways. The 'technical view' is that an environmental shock (bad weather), limited information and import bottlenecks resulted in famine. The 'political view' attributes blame to different actors, depending on who one talks to: the IMF for recommending the sale of strategic food stock; Malawian politicians for selling off the entire food reserve, and making money on the side; complacent government and donor officials; and profiteering traders inflating prices. The truth lies somewhere in a combination of the technical and political views.

In addition to these immediate causes of famine, there are a number of underlying vulnerability factors that left poor Malawians unable to cope with a production shock that was actually less severe than the drought of 1991–1992:

- declining soil fertility and neglect of smallholder agriculture, particularly in remote areas
- deepening poverty that decimated asset buffers (foodstocks, savings)
- weakened informal systems of social protection in poor communities
- the demographic and economic consequences of HIV/AIDS.

Better weather in mid-2003 has been followed by a period of low rainfall. Recent reports describe a country struggling through the lean season, on the brink of another food crisis.

The Zimbabwe situation

In many ways Zimbabwe represents an archetype of a third-world country in which health programmes have been drastically undermined by totalitarian rule. In Chapter 2, Zimbabwe was used as a good example of a country trying to resist the inroads of first-world corporate interests. Its government had stipulated that it would only borrow from the IMF/World Bank up to the extent that repayment on the loans would not exceed 10% of export earnings. We have seen how short-lived this policy was.

As one of many third-world nations, and as one among several in Africa itself, Zimbabwe was in no position to dictate to either the IMF or the first-world banks behind it. If it needed loans, Zimbabwe would have to agree to structural adjustment policies and everything stemming from them. No doubt, had there existed some huge pan-African bloc negotiating as a whole with the IMF, things might have been different, but that was not the case. Second, Zimbabwe, along with South Africa, Zambia and Tanzania, has been among the world leaders in levels of HIV/AIDS prevalence. And, finally, the author's continuing access to health institutions and to health personnel in Zimbabwe has allowed him to document, especially on the basis of the HIV/AIDS epidemic, pivotal issues in the matter of global health promotion. This has been especially valuable in illustrating how intrusive non-medical cultural factors are and, at the same time, how entrenched gender inequalities interfere with health promotion. It is one aim of this chapter to show how IMF funding renders these obstacles to healthcare and promotion more, rather than less, problematical. Consider, for instance, the social position of women, not only or even particularly in Africa, but in many third-world countries.

Disempowerment of women with respect to HIV/AIDS

Lalonde (1974) stated that a very important element of health promotion is empowerment, a process whereby individual people are encouraged to assert their own autonomy and their self-esteem sufficiently to be able to identify their own health agendas, rather than being told what to do or what is good for their health. But any initiative aimed at engendering empowerment must have a focus, and the focus here is on women's lack of empowerment generally in the third world and with special emphasis on promoting safer sex in the face of the HIV/AIDS pandemic.

A number of factors render this concern of pivotal relevance. For instance, the vast majority of the third world's women are poor and lacking in basic education. They can be largely categorised as illiterate women, both married and single, who are perhaps the most disadvantaged of all groups in the world. The author deals here primarily with Zimbabwe, but this is an arbitrary choice, and much the same could be said of Nepal, or many other third-world countries in which he has worked. By definition, empowerment must involve some conflict of social values. This chapter argues that it is possible to empower women, but that prevention programmes have not taken into account the cultural, social and economic constraints, and the male gender roles imposed on most African women, which obstruct the empowerment process. As will also become evident, the fiscal constraints imposed by structural adjustment policies to meet World Bank criteria are rendering the problem even more intractable.

It is generally agreed that men and women in most sub-Saharan African countries are equally at risk of acquiring HIV. With approximately 80% of the risk attributable to heterosexual transmission, prevention, at least in theory, is within the reach of every adult. The prevalence of HIV is currently conservatively estimated at about 25% of the adult, sexually active population infected. In short, this means that about a quarter of working people in Zimbabwe are HIV-positive (Loewnson and Kirkhoven, 1995). The figures relating to Zimbabwe's HIV/AIDS epidemic can be summarised as follows, as of 2000 (Mbizvo, 1997):

- 35% urban HIV prevalence
- 20% rural HIV prevalence
- 1.2 million people HIV-positive
- 200 000 people have developed AIDS
- 90 000 have died of AIDS.

Fiscal considerations, of course, are a major constraint. Because of the continued absence of a preventive vaccine or until therapy recently to cure AIDS, measures for prevention remained the mainstay of Zimbabwean public health promotion strategy. Interventions, such as behavioural change or factors influencing changes in behaviour, such as regular condom use and loyalty to one sexual partner (Mbizvo, 1997), are prominent. Interventions towards HIV prevention are promoted at the clinics, workplaces, in the community, at nightclubs, soccer matches, political rallies and bus stations, within the family and during lunch-breaks at both government and non-government enterprises.

Among social scientists and health professionals, however, there is widespread concern that many women in the developing countries may not have the power to negotiate change for either themselves or their partners (Worth, 1989). Behavioural change that is driven by crisis is difficult and painful for everyone, but modifying behaviour to prevent HIV transmission poses a special challenge to women (Ulin, 1992). It should come as no surprise that in Zimbabwe the focus of women's health needs has tended to be limited to those that are related to pregnancy, childbirth and child health, to the exclusion of women's health in general, in particular sexual health.

Obviously, there are many sources of empowerment, but to promote safer sex would certainly empower women. The promotion of safer sex *per se*, and throughout the country, is what should have priority, but IMF targets only direct money to vertical and regional-specific remit programmes. A health promotion-based initiative would have to converge on two themes, according to Webb (1997): behavioural empowerment and structural empowerment:

> *Behavioural empowerment allows girls and women to have more control over their sexual activity, either through resisting sexual advances or through negotiating safer sex. It is the increase in decision-making ability of the women that renders them less vulnerable to infection as the incidence of unsafe sex is reduced.*

Structural empowerment involves nothing less than the reduction of economic dependence on men and the improvement of women's socio-legal status (Webb, 1997).

Why women are especially vulnerable

Any consideration of a society's sexual health will rely heavily on initiatives directed at women. But this is especially so with HIV/AIDS for four reasons.

- Women in Africa are being portrayed as the 'dangerous victim of the AIDS outbreak'. The devastating level of infection documented on prostitutes is gratuitously interpreted to mean that without them, the epidemic would not be occurring (Ray *et al.*, 1995).
- In comparison with men, women have an increased risk of exposure to HIV infection and increased vulnerability to developing AIDS for reasons related indirectly and directly to their gender.
- Contextual socio-cultural factors, including the following: widowhood, inheritance, polygamy, low power to make decisions in sexual matters and lack of access of information (De Bruyn, 1992).
- Poor diet, poor hygiene, prostitution and the necessity for some students and young women to use sex as an economic resource (exploitation by 'sugar daddies') (Schoepf, 1983).

Ethnological considerations would lead us to believe that women have greater vulnerability. All sexually transmitted diseases (STDs), including AIDS, are transmitted more efficiently from men to women. Research indicates that men appear to pass on HIV more efficiently than women during unprotected vaginal intercourse, making women more likely to be infected by men than for men to be infected by women.

The cultural context in which any health strategy has to operate is crucial. For example, Stein (1990) comments that the success of current HIV prevention strategies among heterosexual couples depends not so much on efficacy as on the strategy's acceptability to the male partner and on the informed co-operation of both partners. The author argues that until women have it within their power to exercise protection independently, the use of condoms as a way of practising safer sex will require women to resort to persuasive or coercive tactics. This alternative may be difficult for many women, especially in the face of economic dependency and societal expectations of a more compliant female role.

Once again, we must turn to anthropology for further contextualising insights. To appreciate the plight of the Zimbabwean women, it is necessary to briefly consider Zimbabwean marital customs. In the societies of Shona and Ndebele, the main purpose of marriage is to produce children for the husband's lineage. In order to secure the right to the children, the husband's family needs to pay a bride price (lobola) and other sums of money to the wife's family. A wife is expected to be obedient to her husband and in-laws, hardworking and respectful. However, the most important requirement is that she be able to bear children. In the author's experience, Zimbabwean societies prefer sons to be born, rather than daughters. Sons are preferred as they can carry on their father's lineage, while daughters are married to other men and do not carry on their father's lineage.

Local culture and HIV prevention

As in many other cultures, the death of a woman's husband in Zimbabwe is invested with huge consequences. Chabal *et al.* (1995, cited in Campbell, 1997) report that childlessness is a source of shame and humiliation, and is reflected in different funeral rites for childless people. These rites are intended to prevent the deceased from returning as a ghost to wreak havoc because of their anger at not having children. As the woman's husband pays lobola for the right to the couple's children, the position of a married woman is severely threatened if she does not bear children. Often, her in-laws and husband will blame her for the infertility. Although the infertility problem may lie with the husband, that possibility is often ignored and not even acknowledged by men. Biased and ignorant views ensure that the woman is almost always blamed for infertility. The husband's family may even send the wife back to her family and demand a refund of the lobola, or demand a female relative as a second wife to bear children in her stead, thereby incurring polygamy. Both partners may resort to sex with other partners to effect a pregnancy, thereby putting both partners at greater risk of contracting HIV. Thus, marriage affects the family relationships of men and women in different ways. A married man remains part of his family of origin all his life, while a wife leaves her family to become part of another one.

This immediately makes it obvious that no real improvement in the situation can be expected unless a long-term view is adopted, featuring the strengthening and furthering of general basic education. But, between 1989 and 1996, Zimbabwe reduced spending on primary schooling by 48% and on secondary education by 31% in order to meet structural adjustment policies criteria. In many rural areas this entailed the outright elimination of access to schooling where such had existed before.

Although the health promotion message is that of empowering women, it is well nigh impossible to begin to attain that goal because of the poverty and gender-related factors that prevail in the everyday life of the women. Moreover, the eradication of those factors requires a political commitment and more use of public funds for education. But HIV prevention strategies can only empower women to a limited extent. Beyond that they will require the co-operation and support of their male counterparts.

Male condoms: culture and consequences

Persuading men to use condoms, especially during recreational sex, has long been reported as difficult in all societies. But some argue that this represents an even greater problem for African men and for a number of cultural reasons. This is especially so if the men are already married. Many studies have pointed out that many people do not enjoy using condoms and prefer to have intercourse without them (Campbell, 1997). Attention has been drawn to the fact that women often have difficulty in negotiating condom use because of the power imbalances between the sexes. The author argues that even when women ask their husbands and partners to use condoms, they often encounter male refusal, are accused of adultery or promiscuity, are suspected of already being infected with HIV or are said to accuse their partners of infidelity (Schoepf, 1983). This view is supported by Wight (1992), who points out that condom use often implies sexual activity outside the primary relationship, or even promiscuity. The limited control that women have in determining their own lives forms part of the social substrate of the current epidemic. The subordination of African women in patrilineal societies places them at a special disadvantage with regard to their ability or willingness to intervene and to reduce their own risk of HIV infection. For many women, faced with divorce or dire poverty, on the one hand, and the risk of HIV infection, on the other, the choice becomes one of social death or biological death (Ray *et al.*, 1995).

Wilson *et al.* (unpublished) argue that studies of sub-Saharan Africa suggest that, although there is a high level of knowledge about HIV transmission, this knowledge has not resulted in effective and appropriate sexual risk reduction practices, specifically condom use. Maposhere *et al.* (1995) revealed that only 38% of Harare men reported condom use. Campbell and Kelly (1995) point to beliefs that it is harmful for a man not to be sexually relieved when he feels the urge. Fears that men will go elsewhere to find sexual relief may prompt women to have sex with their partners in an attempt to ensure sexual fidelity. In this way, a woman's own and her children's economic stability is ensured by her sexual compliance, even within a context where sexual activity outside the relationship is common or even expected.

In many third-world societies, production of offspring is held to be of high importance. Thus, in African societies the greatest deterrent to the use of condoms may be their contraceptive effect. The limited success of family planning programmes in sub-Saharan countries is testimony to the powerful social and cultural constraints on any effort to reduce fertility. Indeed, the resistance of African families to contraception has hindered efforts to prevent vertical transmission of HIV (Ulin, 1992).

In addition, stresses within individual families play a major role. For instance, studies from several sub-Saharan African countries document women's fears of family conflict, economic loss and lowered self-esteem if they advocate condom use (Bledsoe, 1989; Perlez, 1991;

cited in Ulin, 1992). Nonetheless, these women are acutely aware of their own risk of acquiring AIDS and the vulnerability of their children if they should become infected. At the centre of this conflict of values is the condom. For many the condom is not a symbol of reproductive health but of the painful process of negotiating behavioural change.

Even in developed nations, some women feel ambivalent about insisting on condom use. African women with whom this author has discussed the matter often say that, if they do carry male condoms, they feel embarrassment about every stage of condom use. They put their reputation at risk, by buying condoms, carrying them and asking for their use. All these aspects are very difficult for them. Having a condom on one's person indicates a lack of sexual innocence, an unfeminine identity and that of a woman actively seeking sex (Lear, 1995). The author, in speaking with numerous Zimbabwean women, agrees with the view that men will assume that such a woman is cheap and easy, and most probably a prostitute.

Are female condoms the answer?

One solution may be to promote the use of female condoms. The current introduction of female condoms may empower women (Stein, 1990). Since it is used by the woman rather than the man, it gives women greater control over sexual decision-making. Ironically, while empowering women to some degree, it may free men from taking responsibility for their own health (Richardson, 1990). Thus there is a certain ambvalence among women about the real advantages of the female condom. It is interesting to note that, in the first world, the female condom has almost vanished, but, as Burt (2005) pointed out, it is proving to be a godsend to women's empowerment as it gains acceptance in the third world. Of course, it has certain disadvantages when compared with male condoms.

The female condom is much more expensive than the male equivalent and few women can afford it. But research carried out by Ray *et al.* (1995) on commercial sex workers and family planning clinics in both urban and rural areas showed all three groups reacting favourably and even preferring them to the traditional male version. Sex workers are particularly insistent that it is important, recognising the advantage of having more power to negotiate the use of condoms simply by virtue of the exchange relationship between buyer and seller.

However, to the extent that most women lack a voice in sexual decision-making, AIDS prevention campaigns may be overoptimistic in expecting sudden behaviour change. Winters (1997) reports that the government of Zimbabwe and other donor agencies are helping to empower women by selling the female condoms at subsidised prices for women in the lower socio-economic groups. Such categorisation in itself raises problems, of course. Although the female condoms are being sold at subsidised prices, they are not systematically or efficiently distributed across the country. The WHO and other international bodies must play their part in facilitating the availability of female condoms for all women. Surprisingly, it is an enterprise which has not yet attracted a great deal of response from non-governmental organisation aid groups.

STDs as an 'acceptable risk'

A speedy response to STD infection is crucial, and thus an important way of empowering women would be to educate them to seek help in the event of them contracting such an infection. Research indicates that the transmission of HIV is facilitated by genital ulcer disease, which causes lesions and disrupts the mucosal barrier, and this in turn facilitates HIV transmission (Subuga *et al.*, 1990, cited in Pitt *et al.*, 1995). Ray *et al.* (1995) suggest that the link between STDs and AIDS is two-fold. First, the presence of STDs serve as a marker of sexual activity outside the family unit, thus indicating areas where AIDS is likely to spread. Second, in Zimbabwe, nearly half of genital ulcer incidence is caused by chancroid infections in men.

Women experience fewer STD symptoms, and even when they do, they tend to avoid STD care because of stigmatism and because they accept discomfort as part of their reproductive lives. Over 80% of women with STDs receive no care, thus increasing HIV vulnerability (Pitt *et al.*, 1995). Even if women go to clinics, the nurses at the clinics often convey a very judgemental attitude towards them because STDs are regarded as a sign of promiscuity on the woman's part. There is no privacy, and confidentiality is not assured. This, in turn, makes vulnerable women avoid STD treatment, which they need in order to reduce the risk of contracting HIV. Again, this illustrates a real inadequacy in a policy of reducing public spending on general education and directing IMF funding to vertical, interventionist, practices and projects.

In many societies, cultural double standards honour men who have many sexual partners while stigmatising women who have sexual relations outside marriage. Having STDs is almost regarded as a rite of passage into manhood and proof of sexual activity! The author advocates the view that women should be educated about the signs and symptoms of STDs and the importance of seeking early treatment. More research is necessary to examine possible intervention strategies which may develop women's power, increase their ability to negotiate sexual matters and persuade men that the use of condoms is not unmanly. Pitt *et al.* (1995) also argue that the belief that men have rights to multiple sexual partners needs to be challenged, and many health programmes will continue to be only partly effective in changing behaviour until these issues of inequality between the genders are more fully addressed.

The effect of lack of basic education

MacDonald (1998) found that about 30% of a sample of 500 London 16–18-year-old girls had seriously incomplete knowledge of the basic anatomy underlying their sexual health. It is not surprising that in Zimbabwe studies suggest that most women do not know how their reproductive organs work. There are some cultural beliefs that put women more at risk of HIV infection. For example, there is widely held belief that the vagina should be dry, tight and hot for a man to enjoy sex. The herbal ointments that these women use should be discouraged, as they may damage the vaginal wall and open the way for the transmission of HIV and other STDs (Brown *et al.*, 1993). Such mythology can only gain widespread credence in societies in which schools do not widely, and from an early age, address human sexuality as a routine part of the curriculum. Lack of such education also encourages unquestioning acceptance of male dominance values. For instance, in many of these communities the success of a couple's sex life is measured in terms of the amount of pleasure the man receives, and women define their satisfaction by the degree of pleasure they give.

In 1994, Civic and Wilson found that when couples practise dry sex with a condom, there is a very good chance of the condom breaking, thus exposing the couple to a high risk of contracting HIV. Results of the same study suggest that, although individuals may accept handouts of condoms and initiate condom use, they may not use them effectively.

But let us not ignore the existing sources of women's empowerment, for, even in male-dominated societies, women have a certain
degree of autonomy which expresses itself in women's groups. Rural
women have always found strength in informal organisations,
mobilising themselves around specific needs and activities, and using
neighbourhood groups and other informal networks to accomplish
their aims. To quote March and Taggy (1982):

> Women's associations promote confidence, organise leadership and
> resources and thereby create leverage for women, although they may
> not prevent the overall structural authority of men over women, they
> do redistribute power and resources in some very important ways.

Thus we see that women who share common experiences, and face
common risks, can make a conscious decision to take action with the
expectation that the benefits to all will ultimately outweigh the costs.
Through informal associations and networking, African women in the
general population typically rally behind each other to solve numerous
common problems (March and Taggy, 1982). However, Ulin (1992)
argues that this source of strength seems not to have been recognised
and utilised by the policymakers who direct AIDS campaigns.
Women's collective perception of their ability to act as AIDS prevention agents could be a critical determinant of both female and male
behaviour change. But such 'local group autonomy' does not fit in
with privately funded structural adjustment policies initiatives.

Entrenching poverty: a structural adjustment policies bequest

It has been argued throughout this book that structural adjustment
policies often exacerbate, rather than ameliorate, the financing of
health initiatives in third-world countries. Again, the most important
factor governing HIV/AIDS prevention programmes is that of poverty.
This poverty affects the women most because of the lack of economic
opportunities, and the social inequality of women increases their
vulnerability to HIV/AIDS and STDs. During the years 1991–1993 the
economic security of every citizen in Zimbabwe became increasingly
threatened by the introduction of the Economic Structural Adjustment Programme (ESAP). The programme was imposed by the World
Bank on Zimbabwe to repay an IMF loan. Though this programme
aimed to improve the living conditions of the population by making

the economy more productive and competitive, for the great majority of people of low socio-economic status its immediate effects were exactly the opposite (Meursing, 1997).

Sexual health has been even further jeopardised in Zimbabwe by economic recession. That, together with ESAP programmes, has aggravated the transmission and undermined control of HIV infection in Zimbabwe and Africa in two major ways: directly, by increasing the population at risk through increased urban migration, the subsequent impoverishment and women's powerlessness and prostitution; and indirectly, through a decrease in healthcare provision (Sanders and Abdulrahman, 1991).

As is often the case, the forces of nature have also not been co-operative. The economic strain caused by ESAP was compounded by the severe droughts of 1991 and 1992. George and Sabelli (1994) state that, even back then, approximately US $50 000 was leaving Zimbabwe every hour to pay back the IMF loan. Stoneman (1994, cited in George and Sabelli, 1994) commented that, at the behest of the World Bank, Zimbabwe has also turned one of Africa's best healthcare and educational records into a virtual shambles. As one woman put it: '''Health For All by the Year 2000'' is not going to be achieved. Instead, because of ESAP, it will be ''Death For All by the Year 2000''. The élite will not die but they will be very lonely, there will be no one to live with them' (MacDonald, 2005).

Consider just some of the negative impacts so far engendered. Many women can no longer afford hospital births. Children are leaving school early; girls will be the first to be withdrawn from school in order to assist in the home. In Zimbabwe approximately 70% of hospital bed occupancy is HIV-related. The World Bank estimates that the direct hospital costs per Zimbabwean AIDS patient averages US $614. On top of all that, women – once they have become infected – have a shorter survival expectancy than men. There are several reasons for this. Women have less access to healthcare. Unlike men, they engage in numerous activities that do not stop when they are ill; they are also expected to care for their sick husbands or relatives, regardless of their own health. When women are unwell, fewer household members care for them (Barnet and Blackie, 1992). In interviews of Zimbabwean hospital workers, the author was told that often relatives will encourage a man who appears fit and well to leave his AIDS-stricken wife and find another one, with no understanding that he may pass the infection on to another woman.

Any serious attempt at reversing these negative effects must involve policy changes. Clearly, strategies to address the impact of AIDS on women are most likely to be effective if they approach the problem at different levels, working to reverse women's social, economic and legal disadvantage (simultaneously with AIDS) on their lives (Danzier, 1994). This is the complete opposite of the sort of IMF-favoured 'vertical planning'. For example, enhancing opportunities for women's economic independence may require legal and economic reform, and changes in social and educational policy, as well as community programmes for social reform. All of these require more government commitment to public policy initiatives, rather than the blind action of market forces. At the same time, efforts need to be made at the community level to change customs and attitudes which perpetuate women's disadvantages.

A diluted WHO target on HIV/AIDS

The WHO 56th World Health Assembly in Geneva (19–28 May 2003) passed a resolution on 'Global Health Sector Strategy for HIV/AIDS', backing away from re-endorsing its year 2000 strategy, called the 'three-by-five target'. This referred to the aim of ensuring that three million people with AIDS receive anti-retroviral treatment by 2005. Instead, the WHO changed the target's language to 'bearing it in mind' – and this was done at the request of some first-world countries in the European Union (EU). The concern remains that the global fight against HIV/AIDS continues to be grossly underfunded, with the failure to facilitate access to available treatment to millions dying of the disease in Africa and other developing regions. This represents a denial of the fundamental human right to health. India submitted an amendment to the AIDS resolution, calling on countries to increase expenditure on global AIDS programmes, recalling the commitment by all member countries to the UN at the 2001 UN General Assembly Special Session on HIV/AIDS to give US $7–10 billion per year by 2005, but it was not accepted. Non-governmental organisations such as Health GAP, Act UP Paris and other Fund-the-Fund allies advocated a dues-based commitment to full funding of the Global Fund to Fight AIDS, tuberculosis and malaria. However, no explicit language to this effect was forthcoming.

Huge obstacles, linked to the financial interests of the first-world pharmaceutical companies, still remain, as Dyer (2004) reported in the *British Medical Journal*. International health charities have accused George Bush's administration of trying to block developing countries' access to cheap AIDS drugs by questioning the quality of 'three in one' generic combination drugs. At a meeting in August 2004, in Gaborone, Botswana, the US global AIDS co-ordinator, Randall Tobias, said that the WHO's drug pre-qualification programme was not a sufficiently stringent approval process to ensure consistency and quality of fixed-dose combination drugs. He told delegates from national drug regulatory agencies, the pharmaceutical industry and non-governmental organisations that the USA was unwilling to spend the US $15 billion promised in the presidential emergency plan for AIDS relief (PEPFAR) on drugs of unknown quality.

Médecins Sans Frontières and other non-governmental organisations working with AIDS patients in Africa accused the US government of trying to escape the 2001 Doha agreement on affordable drugs (Vass, 2001). The objections raised by Tobias (2003) also threatened implementation of the WTO's August 2003 agreement which specifies how countries with limited or no capacity to manufacture drugs can gain access to cheaper generic medicines. Sharonann Lynch, of the charity Health GAP, said the US government was trying to ensure that the money from the US AIDS relief plan went to brand-name manufacturers: 'These objections make no sense. The generic drugs are bioequivalent compounds, and the WHO pre-qualifications process uses staff from Canadian and European regulatory bodies that the US recognises.' The cheapest generic combination pills cost about US $125 per person per year under a price agreement negotiated with manufacturers by former US President, Bill Clinton. The same combination from brand-name companies costs about US $496 per person per year.

Addressing Congress on 18 March 2004, Mr Tobias, a former chief executive of Eli Lilly, said the US government's objections were motivated by concern for the safety of patients with AIDS: 'We have been reading stories lately about some problems with some drugs around the world, where people with the best of intentions have made acquisitions of drugs that have turned out to not have the consistency, safety, and effectiveness that people had hoped' (US Congressional Record, 19 March 2004).

What is to be done?

The HIV/AIDS pandemic, deeply rooted in so many of the economic, social, cultural, biological and religious customs of humanity, will be with us for some time. But it is not really deniable that it is exacerbated enormously because of the iniquitous exploitation of the third world by the first. Therefore, we have a number of fronts on which to work, such as the following.

• Continued medical research on its epidemiology and other purely clinical aspects.

• Education. Much of the harm done by HIV and other STDs relies on it being immodest to discuss it openly. Children need to know about it and how to avoid it long before puberty. Cautionary advice has a much greater likelihood to be ignored once the hormones get going. Shame and ignorance are the two most potent and effective agents in promoting the suffering, family dislocation, financial ruin, grief and death caused by AIDS.

• It is obvious that abstention works if it is used but it rarely is, or not for long. Condoms for both males and females are much more reliable, whatever religious orthodoxies might preach.

• Respect for human rights is the foundation stone of a psychologically healthy society and a biomedically healthy one as well. That is why health promotion, with its emphasis on empowerment, is so crucial in combating such scourges as AIDS and STDs generally. We have to learn to respect ourselves for only then can we respect one another.

• Internationalism – a situation in which we regard our common global citizenship as of paramount importance – is basic to all of the rest. Such a goal would require a large degree of voluntary investment in some kind of trans-national governance, that will require great imagination, compassion and determination to bring it about. These issues are given some airing in the final chapter of this book.

• The principles of health promotion need to be applied with the same degree of foresight and community involvement in the third world as they are in many first-world nations. The Nepalese epidemiologist, Dr Padan Simkhada, now Research Fellow, Medical School, University of Aberdeen, and recently a delegate to the Bangkok International HIV/AIDS conference, made the point well in an e-mail he sent to the author on 6 August 2004, as follows:

Focusing on prevention of HIV and on expanding access to anti-retroviral treatment for people living with AIDS is critically important to the fight against HIV/AIDS, but alone this strategy is not enough to tackle the problem.

Sustainable and more appropriate prevention and treatment of HIV/ AIDS requires empowering people to act and bring about change in their own terms. Combating HIV/AIDS in developing countries requires more than disease-specific biomedical interventions. It must be linked to broader development strategies. It requires improving the conditions under which people are free to choose safer life strategies and conditions for themselves. For example, at the individual level, better education or better employment makes individuals more likely to protect themselves from contracting HIV. At the same time, improved economic, cultural, political, human rights and social conditions for disempowered or marginalised groups such as migrant workers, improve the effectiveness of HIV/AIDS prevention and treatment programmes.

- Such levels of empowerment must rely heavily on the support of the wealthier nations in a globalised system of international trade and aid regulations.
- Local and community administrations urgently need to address infrastructure issues, such as road and rail transport. It is obvious, from what this author has observed, that even when ARVs and ancillary treatments are available, many third-world people are not within accessible reach of the relevant clinical facilities. To meet these needs, governments would have to forego verticalisation strategies and the levels of priviatisation of healthcare called for by IMF structural adjustment policies and the WTO. But they really have little choice, and pressure needs to be brought by people in first-world societies on their own governments to change their own policies.

References

Barnet T and Blackie P (1992) *AIDS in Africa: its present and future impact.* Bellhaven Press, London.

BBC World Service (2005) Pills, patients and profits. 4 August. Available at BBC World Service archive www.ws.com.documentary. Accessed 1 August 2005.

Bledsoe C (1989) The Cultural Meaning of AIDS and Condoms for Stable, Heterosexual Relations in Africa; recent evidence from the local print. Media paper presented at the IUSSP Seminar on Population Policy in sub-Saharan Africa, 'Drawing on International Experience', Kinshasa.

Brown JE, Ayowa OB and Brown RC (1993) Dry and tight sexual practices and potential AIDS risk in Zaire. *Social Science and Medicine.* **37**: 989.

Burt K (2005) Whatever happened to the Femidom? *Guardian.* 23 August.

Campbell T (1997) How can psychological theory help to promote condom use in sub-Saharan African developing countries? *Journal of the Royal Society of Health.* **117**: 186–91.

Campbell T and Kelly J (1995) How can psychology theory help promote condom use in sub-saharan African developing countries. *Journal for the Royal Society of Health.* **117**(3): 211–14.

Chabal T, Campbell T and Sheth S (1995) Issues raised in a counselling support group for HIV positive people in Zambia. *Journal of the British Association of Counselling.* **6**: 211–14.

Chronic Poverty Report (2004–05) What should be done about chronic poverty? Chronic Poverty Research Centre, University of Manchester, Manchester.

Civic D and Wilson D (1994) Dry sex in Zimbabwe and implications of condom use. *Social Science and Medicine.* **42**: 91–8.

Danzier R (1994) The social impact of HIV/AIDS in developing countries. *Social Science and Medicine.* **39**: 905–9.

De Bruyn M (1992) Women and AIDS in developing countries. *Social Science and Medicine.* **34**: 249–62.

Dyer O (2004) Bush accused of blocking access to cheap AIDS drugs. *BMJ.* **328**: 783.

Flick F (2003) World Trade Organization finally agrees cheap drugs deal. *BMJ.* **327**: 517.

George S and Sabelli F (1994) *Faith and Credit: the World Bank's secular empire.* Penguin, London.

Lalonde M (1974) *Perspectives on the Health of Canadians.* Government of Canada Publications, Ottawa.

Lear D (1995) Sexual communication in the age of AIDS: the construction of risk and trust among young adults. *Social Science and Medicine.* **4**: 1311–23.

Loewenson R and Kirkhoven A (1995) Socio-Economic Impact of AIDS Issues and Options. Study prepared for Sida, Sweden. Executive Summary.

Lovich R (2004) *HIV/AIDS at a Glance.* Save the Children, Washington, DC.

MacDonald T (1998) *Rethinking Health Promotion: a global approach.* Routledge, London.

MacDonald T (2005) *Third World Health: hostage to first world wealth.* Radcliffe Publishing, Oxford.

Maposhere C, Manyeya S and Zhuwau T (1995) Male Condom Accessibility and Availability within Health Centres in Zimbabwe. Study prepared for the National Aids Co-ordination Programme. Department of Health, Harare, Zimbabwe.

March KS and Taggy R (1982) *Women's Informal Associations and the Organizational Capacity for Development.* Monograph Series No. 5, Rural Development

Committee, Centre for International Studies, Cornel University, Ithaca, New York.

Mbizvo M (1997) Towards a Strategy for HIV Prevention in Zimbabwe: what interventions work? Symposium report, University of Zimbabwe.

Meursing K (1997) *A World of Silence: living with HIV in Matebeleland, Zimbabwe.* KIT Publications, Amsterdam.

Perlez J (1991) AIDS outweighed by the desire to have a child. *New York Times.* 26 April.

Pitts M, Bowman M and McMaster H (1995) Reactions to repeated STD infections: psychological aspects and gender issues in Zimbabwe. *Social Science and Medicine.* 40(a): 1299–304.

Ray S, Bassett M, Maphoshere C, Manangasira P, Nicolette JD, Macheleano R and Moyo J (1995) Acceptability of the female condom in Zimbabwe: positive but male-centred responses. *Journal of Reproductive Health Matters.* 5: 68–79.

Richardson D (1990) AIDS education and women: sexual and reproductive issues. In: P Aggleton, P Davies and G Hart (eds) *AIDS: individual, cultural and policy dimensions.* Flamer Press, London.

Sanders D and Abdulrahman S (1991) AIDS in Africa: the implications of economic recession and structural adjustment. *Health Policy and Planning.* 6: 157–65.

Schoepf BG (1983) Women, AIDS and economic crisis in Central Africa. *Central Journal of African Studies.* 3: 662–5.

Stein B (1990) Women and contraception in developing societies. In: P Azzleton, P Davis and G Hart (eds) *AIDS: individual and cultural policy dimensions.* Flamer Press, London.

Stoneman C. Cited in George S and Sabelli F (1994) *Faith and Credit: The World Bank's Secular Empire.* Penguin, London.

Subuga A *et al.* Cited in Pitts M, Bowman M and McMaster H (1995) Reactions to repeated STD infections: psychological aspect and gender issues in Zimbabwe. *Social Science and Medicine.* 40(9): 1299–304.

Tobias R (2003) www.law.fsu.edu/WebNews/archives/issue29/Page2. Accessed 22 January 2006.

Ulin P (1992) African Woman and AIDS: negotiating behavioural change. *Social Science and Medicine.* 34: 63–73.

UNAIDS (2003) Joint UNAIDS /Parliamentary forum on AIDS 2003. *Chronic Poverty Report 2004/5.* Institute for Development Policy and Management. University of Manchester.

Vass A (2001) WTO relaxes rule on drug patents. *BMJ.* 326: 1146.

Webb D (1997) *HIV and AIDS in Africa.* Pluto Press, London.

Wight D (1992) Impediments to safer heterosexual sex: a review of research with young people. *AIDS Care.* 4: 11–21.

Wilson D, Nyathi B and Nhariwa M (unpublished) A Community Level AIDS Prevention Programme among Sexually Vulnerable Groups and the Population in Bulawayo, Zimbabwe.

Winters J (1997) Social marketing of condoms (female too) gets going (again). *AIDS Analysis Africa*. **7**: 6.

Worth D (1989) Sexual decision making and AIDS: why condom promotion among vulnerable women is likely to fail. *Studies in Family Planning*. **20**: 297.

Chapter 6

What are the solutions?

What's new?

Having indicated in the Preface why the present situation is unique in human history, and having agreed that most of the serious problems we face are a consequence of trade between the first and third worlds being controlled by capitalism and the dictates of neo-liberal economics, do we have any right to face the future with optimism? We do. In the 1980s the average person was much more aware of issues such as air pollution and racism than they were in the 1950s. Even primary school syllabi widely reflected these concerns. Today we have moved far beyond that. Not a week goes by without detailed accounts in the media of global warming, the irresponsibility of oil producers and the politics involved, environmental sustainability, rising water levels and so on. There is very little likelihood that we will allow ourselves to sleepwalk into irreversible assaults on the environment or genocide. But, while we have cause for optimism, we have no cause for complacency. Action is called for at all levels: individual, community and political.

Recognising that to address any of the issues that follow in detail in one chapter of a book is a tall order, three broad areas of solutions are indicated, as follows:

- approaches to environmental sustainability
- community organisation
- political alternatives.

Each of these categories is so broad, however, that they will have to be subdivided.

Approaches to environmental sustainability

This is an enormous topic in itself and, thankfully, one with which a great deal of active engagement is taking place. Let us start by considering our options with respect to fuels. It is clear that we must move away from non-renewable sources before they begin to run out and, at the same time, we have to avoid using those sources whose combustion produces greenhouse gases. Research on alternatives has been so intense over the past 20 years that Chandler (2004), writing in the *New Scientist*, asserts that the technologies to deliver clean and sustainable energies already exist. What is temporarily stopping us from advancing on that front is politics – plus vested interests such as the automobile lobby and various oil industries. There is also a wide-based feeling that alternative sources of energy, such as biomass, wind, wave and tide, are too theoretical and remote from realisation. But a raft of research studies, some even financed by the oil companies, suggest otherwise.

If this view is correct, the pay-offs in terms of human rights, health and fair trade would be enormous. No more massive tax-supported subsidies for oil exploration and extraction, no more cultivation of war in the Middle East (which is estimated to have 65% of the world's oil reserves) and no more extravagant carbon dioxide emissions. The only losers would be large corporations and their stock-holders, whereas most other people would benefit. It would certainly save Alaska, because one key provision of George W Bush's 2004 Energy Bill would allow oil drilling in one of Alaska's wildlife reserves. If this went ahead, environmentalists claim that its impact on the region's fragile ecosystem would be disastrous and would have environmental consequences well beyond Alaska's shores.

A recent study (Chandler, 2004) showed that there exist 15 suitable alternative technologies already. Even without drastic changes, applying present technologies can double the average fuel efficiency of cars, and can heat and light homes and public buildings at a much lower cost and with greatly reduced carbon dioxide emissions (Pacala and Socolow, 2004). Pacala and Socolow (2004) claim that even though some alternatives such as hydrogen-fuelled cars themselves involve environmental problems adopting just a few of these could stabilise levels of global greenhouse gases in the atmosphere by the year 2050. There are many other such studies widely accessible on the internet.

Use of biomass

One alternative which has recently attracted much attention is the idea of using biomass. Radford (2005), Science Editor of the *Guardian* newspaper, pointed out that the biomass issue merits serious attention. Biomass is easily produced and can be made from straw, woodchips, willow coppice, mildewed grain, chicken litter and sewage sludge. According to Radford (2005), it could provide a significant amount of the nation's energy needs. He then explains that a million hectares of British countryside could be used for sources of biomass, helping to create a cleaner and greener Britain, and avoid 20 million tonnes of carbon dioxide emissions a year. These figures were backed up by a government report in October 2005.

Such an action, if carried out now, would run up against local council ordinances. Before anything can happen, the government has to rethink development rules. It also needs to provide coherent advice, if not financial help, to potential developers. Sir Ben Gill, a former president of the National Farmers' Union, said that government rules devised 50 years ago to control atmospheric pollution need to be modified for biomass to be produced. He went on to say that another critical barrier is popular ignorance about the quantity of what is available, how to source it, the relevant transformation technologies, forms of biomass and about safety issues. There is also widespread ignorance about the flexibility of biomass and how it could be fitted into modern technologies. Straw bales and woodchips, like coal and oil, produce carbon dioxide emissions. But coal and oil draw on a reserve 'energy bank' laid down about 300 million years ago. Biomass, on the other hand, withdraws and pays back into the the planet's 'current account' and, in the long term, makes no difference to levels of greenhouse gases causing climate change and global warming.

New computer-controlled furnaces and reactors already exist to attract fuel, heat and electricity from biomass. Schemes have also been developed to exploit the locked up energy more efficiently. Plans even exist for financing such enterprises. According to Sir Ben Gill, 'There is such a lot of information available about it, that people lose their way in it!' (Radford 2005) These problems are discussed in a recent Department for Environment, Food and Rural Affairs (DEFRA) report to promote discussion and debate about the matter. The report argues for new ways of thinking about energy use, noting that power stations smaller than the present ones and sited near towns could provide both heat and electricity with huge savings. Sir Ben went on to say, 'We waste enough heat from old power stations to heat the whole country one and a half times over. We are a country concerned about climate change and the use of fossil fuel, yet we're wasting all of that energy. The take-home message has to be that, instead of being tomorrow's fuel, biomass should be today's fuel' (Radford, 2005).

Naturally, none of the proposed solutions with biomass is problem-free. Monbiot (2004) argues that the adoption of biofuels would be a humanitarian and environmental disaster. His reasoning, briefly, is that to sustain prevailing rates of fuel consumption by motorists would require so much acreage of land for the biomass crops that widespread famine would ensue. He notes that, since car drivers are much wealthier than non-drivers, the former would simply seize the land they needed to produce fuel for their vehicles. But that, of course, assumes no behaviour change in people and communities faced with palpable disaster, a most unlikely scenario.

How feasible is use of hydrogen?

What about powering cars with hydrogen? At the simple level, it looks good because the only emission would be water vapour. The problem so far has been that producing the hydrogen in the quantities required would be environmentally costly. Of course, as Brown (2004) points out, we could derive the hydrogen from nuclear power stations. This, though, is not really an agreeable solution.

Whatever is said about the environmental advantages of nuclear power, scientists have yet to solve the problem of what to do with spent fuel rods. They remain dangerously radioactive for at least 250 000 years. Until we solve that problem, conservative instincts suggest that we use nuclear power sparingly, if at all. Indeed, it is not even truly sustainable because reserves of uranium will only last for another 125–150 years (Toke, 2004), so by using nuclear power we would, again, be living off our savings and not the interest. It is also highly risky, especially if a nuclear power station were either attacked or destroyed in some natural calamity. Such power stations would also be a natural target for people searching for material for aggressive military purposes.

Addressing a meeting of the World Nuclear Association, held in London in September 2004, Professor Paul Kruger of California's Stanford University presented an alternative view, telling delegates that a combination of the need to cut carbon dioxide emissions, increasingly expensive oil and the growth in the world's vehicle numbers, means that hydrogen is the only fuel that can easily meet those needs. He believes that hydrogen will soon be produced by combining renewables such as wind and solar power and a small number of nuclear power stations designed to produce hydrogen with surplus electricity.

Although a handful of buses in the UK already run on hydrogen fuel, and given that BMW has designed a dual petrol/hydrogen engine, we are still faced with the problem of how to produce enough hydrogen to replace oil altogether. But that is surely a challenge to scientists, a project worth working on while limited nuclear power is used in the meantime to generate the hydrogen required.

Professor Kruger went on to say that making slightly larger nuclear power stations would generate enough surplus electricity to run hydrogen production cleanly. It could also be sold to a national network of hydrogen filling stations for fuel cells in cars. Advisers to President Bush are so convinced that dual electricity and hydrogen production is the way forward that the US Department of Energy has decided to construct a demonstration nuclear reactor to produce hydrogen in the state of Idaho. Hans Forsstrom, from the European Commission, has said that the EU was also considering the use of high-temperature non-nuclear reactors to produce hydrogen. He claims that this idea has a huge potential. Klaus Sheuerer of BMW asserts that the firm already has produced a car that could run on either hydrogen or petrol. He said that the long-term transition to hydrogen as a source of energy is an absolute necessity. We are confident that the solution is at hand, reports Brown (2004).

It is hugely satisfying that none of this is particularly remote or theoretical. For instance, most of the foregoing commentators assume that there will be no social or behavioural changes and that the private transport market will simply continue to grow at the rate it has been. Even the problems those people anticipate (and they assume them all to be resolvable in time) would become much less through fairly rudimentary changes in the way that we organise our transport. With any kind of rational planning, should we not be governed by neo-liberal finance, public transport will become the order of the day and the demand for private vehicles (and all of the infrastructure associated therewith) will shrink. Similarly, more enlightened forms of town planning should reduce the need for such enormous power needs. Also, there are alternatives to nuclear power at hand.

Other renewable sources of energy

Solar heating of housing and other buildings is a present and realistic option, even in the UK. The author is at present modifying his own home to accommodate solar heating. The building is an old stone cottage, not at all designed with solar power in mind, which means that it has to be done rather inefficiently. But it can be done and will even cost less to run than conventional methods. By use of currently available technologies, even aircraft could be rendered much less environmentally destructive. But, again, who is to say that we will not elaborate a variety of alternatives to their present widespread use.

Also much more feasible than is widely realised is the potential for the use of renewables such as wind, wave and tide. A mass of up-to-date-material on these is available on the internet and, moreover, is more current than any book can be. For instance, Wind Energy (www.bwea.com/ukwed/statuso705.html) states in its July 2005 report that the UK wind farms alone will, by 2007, be producing enough energy to power 25% of all of the homes in London. The potential for the use of wind has hardly been measured, let alone exploited. Similarly, we are told that studies suggest that the marine environment on the UK coasts stores enough energy in the form of heat, current, waves and tides to meet total worldwide demand for power several times over. Two of the most significant forms around the UK are marine currents, caused by tidal effects, thermal and salinity differences, and waves generated by the action of the winds blowing over the surface of the water (www.bwea.com/marine/resource.html). Wave power potential is also immense. Its global power potential has been estimated to be of the same order of magnitude as current world electrical energy consumption.

Ubuntu: one idea of community organisation

The idea of 'community' as a complete and flexible mechanism for accommodating social survival and social definition seems to have been basic to human cultural evolution. It has virtually only been since the development of capitalism, and the social relations to which it has given rise, that competition in pursuit of individual achievement has been a dominant social feature. The emphasis on individual self-actualisation promotes competition between the individuals in a community rather than co-operation. In that way, much of the first world has gradually lost touch with the concept of community. It therefore might be worth going further back into the history of our social origins to discover what we have lost.

In this regard the third world, and especially Africa (from which the human race is said to have sprung), can teach us a lot. The case is well put by Professor Mogobe Ramose (1999) in his book, *African Philosophy Through Ubuntu*. Professor Ramose describes the concept of Ubuntu as applying (with local variations) over all African societies and as underwriting the entire African experience. It undergirds a co-operative way of life, based on widely extended family relationships that have sustained social development reasonably free from inter-group warfare. It has been characterised rather by an emphasis on negotiated solution of conflict situations by imaginative integrationist strategies as opposed to total conquest and seizure of territory. He argues that this was only subdued under the European imperial idea of the 'right of conquest', which ultimately forced the African people into the money economy. His book is, I suggest, a valuable resource in reinterpreting the theme of community.

The People's Health Movement

In the first world there has emerged in recent years a wider popular appreciation of community as an alternative source of social development, and there are many examples of it, especially relating to education and healthcare. One of the most vibrant of these is the People's Health Movement (PHM). The reader has already seen how the noble aims of the WHO's HFA 2000 were sidetracked in the late 1980s by the demands of neo-liberal globalised finance. The WHO, for various reasons, has found itself unable to resist these pressures and, accordingly, the PHM came into being. It is a splendid example of community empowerment and action.

So far the PHM has held two international meetings, called People's Health assemblies (PHAs). PHA1 was held at Dacca in Bangladesh in 2000 and PHA2 was held in Cuenca, in Ecuador, in July 2005. PHA1 had as its goal the revitalisation of the aims of Alma Ata, as described in Chapter 1, namely bringing about primary healthcare for all. Those aims remain in place, of course, but at PHA2 they were refined and specific community action groups set up. PHA2 was the culmination of five years of planning by a global steering group, as well as by the active involvement of various PHM members throughout the world.

The Cuenca gathering brought together delegates from a wide range of civil society organisations, non-governmental organisations, social activists, health professionals and so forth. It comprised more than 1500 people drawn from 168 countries. This account of the event is drawn largely from a report by Smith (2005), a student at the Albert Einstein School of Medicine in New York and Editor of *Social Medicine Portal*.

The Assembly was organized into two major parallel plenary sessions each morning and six tracks of workshops every afternoon. Of special significance also, is the fact that on the same site, but during the previous week, the International People's Health University (IPHU) had also been held. It attracted about 60 students seeking information and training in the sorts of activism which they could fruitfully apply in their home communities. It was characterized by morning lectures on practical aspects of community health activism, followed by afternoon meetings of small groups dealing with specific issues, such as: health and trade, health rights of indigenous people, women's health issues, the patenting of pharmaceuticals and seed varieties, etc. This author also was privileged to attend the IPHU sessions. The morning sessions were in both Spanish and English, with simultaneous translations, while the afternoon small-group sessions, were in one or the other.

The levels of spontaneous cooperation (e.g. people volunteering to act as translators at a moment's notice) reflected the intense commitment and idealism of the participants. A conference daily newspaper, The Pinjara Daily Alert was even put together by a volunteer team of journalists and had the important function of feeding directly into the normal Ecuadorean media, as well as internationally. PHA2 hence had a high profile and delegates were welcomed warmly on the streets of Cuenca as they made their way to and from sessions. It was this author's experience, and that of fellow delegates, that shop keepers, taxi drivers, all sorts of people, frequently bombarded one with questions about PHM and with accounts of their own community health problems. In keeping with this spirit, the PHA2 culminated in a massive march through the city streets. The atmosphere was strongly upbeat with a great deal of spontaneous local involvement and encouragement. That gathering was addressed by Aleida Guevara, daughter of the famous Ché, and a Cuban pediatrician in her own right.

The People's Health Movement is certainly a part of the solutions to the problems raised in Chapter 1 and a potent example of the power of community action. For many of the US students to the IPHU, it was the first time that they had been out of their country and their first serious contact with alternative ways of looking at global politics. Through conversations with them, one came to appreciate the problems that they must face at home, along with the many great strengths that underlie American social and political history. The conference benefited enormously from their vigour, organisation, innovation and commitment, and strongly illustrated the silliness of the levels of anti-Americanism that one often encounters in progressive circles in the UK and elsewhere. As far as community action is concerned, America must be a crucial part of the equation.

The importance of the US contribution

It seems obvious that we must do everything possible to support American voices denied adequate access to the media in their own country. They need a much more open forum so that, instead of reacting on a reflex of fear and xenophobia to international issues, they have a better opportunity to discuss their concerns about health-care, job security, social equity and so on. We in Europe need to be much more pro-active in opening our media to them in areas so far not dominated by Fox News and the Rupert Murdoch media empire, etc. We cannot afford to remain passive in the face of first-world governments outside the USA having their media brought under the control of capitalism. All these issues need to be thrashed out first at small community level and between communities worldwide. We are all affected and health issues are only one symptom of a much wider problem.

Modern methods of communication – computers, e-mail, tele-conferencing – have been immensely liberating and the US contributions in that arena are indispensable. For instance, even totalitarian regimes seem largely unable to seriously interfere with, or even censor, e-mail. The author has spoken to a number of computer experts about this, but has received no fully satisfactory account of why it is so difficult to monitor. Suffice to say, my research has over the years involved sending and receiving e-mail from medical people in various otherwise sinister dictatorships and even from Rwanda and the Côte d'Ivoire at the height of military conflict and mass murder in those countries. This augurs well for future developments because we are rapidly reaching the situation in which many third-world communities have some computer access. International access to the internet is foreseeable. Never previously in human history has the international exchange of information and ideas been so easy, and it will increase. One obvious reason that many exploited third-world people have in the past remained so passive is that they simply did not know how grossly disadvantaged they were. We must not underestimate the liberation potential of communication developments.

Community health impact assessment

Another recent development harnessing community health has been the idea of health impact assessment (HIA). The idea was first developed in first-world urban contexts as a way of preventing adverse effects on the health of urban communities by allowing firms free rein in setting up commercial enterprises. Under HIA regulations, companies could not be granted a licence to proceed until an independent health monitoring group had carried out an investigation as to the extent that the local population would be affected by factors such as noise, atmospheric pollution, views of local residents and impact on local employment. Only when agreement had been reached between the HIA group and the proposed business, guaranteeing that the local people would not be adversely affected, could the project be considered further.

We need, as a matter of some urgency, to make HIAs part of the international agenda as quickly as possible. This is strongly suggested by several contributors (O'Keefe and Scott-Samuel, 2002), who state 'Health impact assessments can and should aim to provide tools that can capture the most deep-seated, systematic and global economic and environmental crimes in which humankind is complicit'. For instance, all that has been said in earlier chapters about structural adjustment policies or about 'vertical', as opposed to 'horizontal', planning needs consideration. Both these methods of approach protect the first world, but often bring about ecological damage in the third world of such a scale as to undermine health to a grotesque degree.

Setting up the framework for such international HIAs would require a much more radical approach than G8 or WTO summits can possibly provide. In fact, the matter cannot be based on arguments of relative costs to the governments involved. It is an essential and therefore has to be done without financial preconditions. Once we establish, through international meetings of the health experts, what must be done, we can then sit down and work out what participating nations need to contribute financially. The banks and corporations become 'service purveyors', but they cannot call the shots or determine ahead of time what might be in it for their first-world stockholders. Consider what has been done already.

International Association for Impact Assessment and HuIA

The International Association for Impact Assessment (IAIA) was established in 1980 to co-ordinate the efforts of researchers, practitioners and various users of HIAs in different parts of the world and therefore often finds itself advising on third-world health issues. It seeks to:

- develop approaches and practices for comprehensive and integrated HIA; it thus does not confine itself to individual projects in various countries, but takes into account their total community impact
- improve assessment techniques for wide practical application
- promote public understanding and involvement in what they are doing and in setting targets
- share their findings and publications.

The IAIA identifies itself as the leading global authority in the use of HIA for decision-making regarding policies and programmes. It believes the assessment of the environmental, social, economic, cultural and health implication of government or international proposals to be a critical contribution to sustainable development. For more information, consult http://iaia.org. This site was updated on 30 July 2004.

An even more effective initiative for trying to anticipate what the health impact of some international trading or commercial proposal will be is considered by human impact assessment in states (HuIA). This includes both health impact assessment and social impact assessment. The two, of course, are often inextricable. HuIA was initiated in Finland and famously applied in the elaboration of the Finnish Healthy Cities Network. Started in 1993, HuIA has recently been developing strategic prediction tools for global use in sustainable health. For more information, consult http://stakes.fi/sva/huia/huianstates.htm.

This seems a very tall order, but unless we set HIA criteria, as established by health experts and in consultation with the recipient communities, we are lost. The gap between rich and poor is still widening with respect to such human rights as health, education and access to pure water – basically 'human dignity' – and that is because we are treating the problems as ones that have to be solved in the context of business and corporate interests. Of course, many people (usually those in no danger of personal environmental threats to their own dignity) refer to the 'business model' as 'realistic'. Altruism, by that measure, is more often than not 'unrealistic'. But if we allow ourselves to live with that view of reality, we are guaranteeing more wars, more environmental disasters and an early end to our existence.

That is why the serious and systematic application of HIA globally to trade and all other international transactions is 'radical'. It need not involve major revolutionary upheavals and large-scale war. As explained in the rest of this chapter, we should be able to avoid that. There just needs to be a major revolutionary upheaval in our thought processes, an enterprise eminently worth pursuing to prolong civilised values and the pleasures of life.

Political alternatives

Reference was made in Chapter 1 to what was referred to as the 'Cuba phenomenon'. This was in the context of Cuba's exceptionally good healthcare system despite its relative poverty compared with other nations. In other words, Cuba somehow seems to have developed a system under which its health as a nation is unrelated to its wealth. It has continued to lead in this respect, and to contribute enormously to the development of high-tech medical research, despite the increasing severity of the US blockade of the island. The details of this are set out in full in other books by the author (MacDonald, 1984, 1998, 2000, 2005), but, suffice to say, Cuba has achieved its remarkable health statistics (as validated by the WHO, UNESCO and other UN bodies) through developing an extraordinarily complete system of community medicine, based on having available one specialist-trained family doctor for every 310 people, backed up by universally accessible polyclinics and provincial hospitals.

We know that Cuba is a totalitarian society, although after having lived and worked there for six years after the revolution, I have to say it is like no other totalitarian country in which I have served! We also know that modern Cuba traces its history back to January 1959, when revolutionary forces led by Fidel Castro, and which had been fighting for six years, finally triumphed. They overthrew the dictator Fulgencia Batista (who fled to Florida) and proceeded to change Cuba from a typically backward Latin American country, with high rates of illiteracy and ill health, to its present condition. Not only are its health statistics among the best in the world, it has an adult literacy rate of 94% (last measured by UNESCO in 1994), it has a highly developed educational system and an inclusive pre-school system for children below the age of six years. Tertiary education is free for students who meet the tough academic criteria for university entrance (MacDonald, 1998).

Not only does Cuba provide itself handsomely with healthcare staff but, from 1968 onward, it has been sending doctors abroad to help set up and run health services in other third-world countries. Wherever the author worked in the third world, he kept hearing laudatory remarks about visiting teams of Cuban doctors, nurses and ancillary health workers. Space does not permit more than a passing reference to their pioneering work in genetic medicine, successful elaboration of vaccines for meningococcic meningitis Type B, breakthroughs in advanced cardiac surgery and successful treatment for retinitis pigmentosis.

Despite the most intense efforts of the USA to isolate Cuba and undermine it, and its success in bringing the EU nations into line behind its hostile designs on Cuba, Cuba still keeps hitting the medical headlines with its health breakthroughs. In May 2005, for instance, it was able to announce significant progress in developing an immunisation against cholera. In 1997 Cuba established a medical school called the Latin American School of Medicine. Cuba already has 19 medical schools, but this one was built for the sole purpose of training medical students from other third-world countries (particularly from Latin America) so that they could then return home and practise in their own communities. In July 2005, the first cohort of 400 doctors graduated. In total, the school has more than 1600 students.

The US government is anxious to destroy the Cuban regime, and whatever one might say about this being prompted by a love for Western-style democracy, one would have to ask why the USA is not equally intent on subverting various larger Latin American governments with somewhat casual attitudes towards torture and other violations of human rights and most of whose children do not receive either adequate healthcare or schooling. One cannot but suspect that Cuba's real offence has been to arrive at a political system that allows it to offer such good social services without becoming enmeshed in the neo-liberal financial debt-traps of capitalism. If we are really interested in finding solutions to the problems that were identified in Chapter 1, establishing meaningful medical and educational links with Cuba would seem to be a step forward without necessarily constituting an endorsement of totalitarianism.

Trans-national mediation of equity

The UN was established before the end of World War II to oversee equity between nations in such a way as to prevent war. Indeed, it is of no small interest to note that, under the UN Charter, waging war against another country is the worst of international crimes. Iraq and all of its attackers are signatories to that Charter. The UN is an incredibly ambitious project, but can it work given that any nation state in it can refuse to co-operate in its endeavours should those not meet the competitive economic needs of that nation? For instance, Kofi Annan, the present Secretary General of the UN, can shout and plead for other nations to send peace-keeping forces to Darfur to mediate a settlement with Sudan. But if none of the nations approached find it convenient to send such troops, they will not be sent. At present, that conflict is being mediated by a ludicrously small contingent of African Union forces which can neither forestall attacks, rape and pillage by Sudanese forces, nor even help the victims. Meanwhile, attempts to consider the issue at the UN General Assembly are stalled for weeks on such issues as to whether what is happening meets with the definition of 'genocide'. Events in the Republic of the Congo are even worse. There, UN peace-keepers have even been accused of rape, murder and other crimes. This is grist for the mill of much of the US media, which has mounted a campaign of vilification of the UN. Before considering why this has happened, it is worth pointing out that 'UN peace-keepers' are not interviewed, trained or selected by the administrative body in New York, headed by Kofi Annan, but by the country supplying them.

One might ask why the media, especially the US media, should be so insistent in its antagonism towards the UN, as surely their reporters understand the situation. But one only needs to ask who, on the whole, owns and controls most of the first-world media? It tends to be the same people and groupings that control the large multi-national corporations which benefit so handsomely from the skewed trading imbalances characterising globalised commerce.

At the beginning of August 2005, President Bush nominated John Bolten as US Ambassador to the UN. There was such strong opposition to the appointment within the USA itself, that President Bush pushed through the nomination during the summer recess. The reason for this opposition by many thoughtful Americans was that they were aware of John Bolten's barely disguised animus against the UN and his opposition to Kofi Annan. For these reasons, the appointment was regarded with apprehension by global health watchers throughout the world. Bolten did not wait long – three weeks, in fact, to show his true colours. October 2005 was to be the 60th Annual Report of the UN and it had been intended that the Report would demonstrate that the gap in health, wealth and human rights between the first and third worlds had widened significantly over the previous decade. The Report argued that that this increase in poverty posed a growing threat to stability.

On 26 August 2005, Under-Secretary General for the UN Department of Economic and Social Affairs, Jose Antonio Campo, stated that the 2005 Report will focus on the international aspects of inequality, a decision reached by 191 member nations of the UN more than two years ago and on which over 100 of those countries have been actively involved in gathering data. It sounds alarm over the deepening disparities in health, education and economic participation between the first- and third-world countries. According to the UN press release of 25 August 2005, 'Increasing poverty and the growing schism between the haves and have-nots will breed violence and terror if not reversed. This must include addressing economic asymmetries both within and between countries.' At present, 80% of the world's domestic product belongs to the one billion people of the first world, while the remaining 20% is shared by the five billion people of the third world. This, of course, is largely a legacy of economic neo-liberalism and the current methods of monitoring international trade. Jose Antonio Campo went on to note that this Report comes 10 years after the 1995 Copenhagan World Summit for Social Development, where governments (including the UK and the USA) pledged to confront social challenges and to place people at the centre of development proposals. Focusing exclusively on economic growth as a developmental strategy appears to be ineffective (UN, 2005).

What has been John Bolten's response to this report? He has demanded that it largely be scrapped. In other words, he is saying that the judgement of 191 other nations, elaborated over years of hard work, must give way to one nation's views after three weeks of analysis. His comments were summarised in a front page article by Usborne in *The Independent* of 26 August 2005. Usborne states that John Bolten wants to scupper the UN's global strategy with 750 amendments, even though the Report had been approved by Kofi Annan. In particular, the USA would delete any reference to the UN's millennium goals on poverty, disease and inequity. He also wants to eliminate the provision calling on nuclear powers to speed up disarmament, to remove agreed targets on foreign aid to third-world countries, to eliminate provisions to halt global warming and to delete any references at all to the International Criminal Court, the world's only permanent war crimes court. Most interesting, in view of what we have already discussed with respect to the WTO and its powers, Bolten wants to restrict third-world countries from joining the WTO. By way of additions, he wishes to highlight and amplify passages dealing with terrorism and the spreading of democracy. Usborne ends his report with the rhetorical question: 'With Bush's man installed as US Ambassador to the UN, is this the end of diplomacy?'

These problems are bound to arise with the UN as presently constituted. Its stated aim is to mediate international equity, peace and human rights, but how can it do so when the individual nation state can reject its proposals? There surely has to be some kind of transnational authority, which would have to be democratically elected internationally – preferably by citizens rather than governments – which could legitimately call on the resources of member nations to mediate discrepancies in basic human rights. Such an agency, instead of being composed of nations, could comprise delegates from physical geographic regions which are likely to share many of the same environmental hazards and assets. This would then render possible the solution of the present injustices inflicted by WTO trading rules. Such a system would allow an emphasis on fair trade as opposed to free trade by monitoring trade within regions. In health terms, it would greatly facilitate the garnering of resources at local level in fighting disease, organising universal access to reliable and safe water supplies and so forth. Regional HIAs could be used to referee or modify large-scale financial involvements.

Many more idealist thinkers would like to see the emergence of internationalism, a global government of some sort, and an end to feelings of national loyalty. Perhaps that will eventually happen at some future time. But our concern in this book is the search for more immediate solutions to the problems that face us. The concept of 'nation' has been with us for a long time and is inextricably tied in with our mores, arts, culture and religious tendencies. For it to suddenly vanish – not that there is any likelihood that such a thing could be realistically organised – would represent a serious loss and a source of lasting social disorientation.The whole idea of 'solutions' so far discussed has addressed only a few options in a few categories. It is intended to provide a springboard for thought and action and not a complete list of recipes, and there are many issues left out. For a fuller account of this issue, the reader is referred to Chapter 14 of *Third World Health: Hostage to First World Wealth* (MacDonald, 2005).

Is capitalism actually an option?

Much of the health data already discussed in this book suggests that the sort of radical change required in the first world in order to expedite global health must of necessity be inimical to capitalism. How true is this? It is worthwhile now to see how it ties in with sustainability arguments.

There is first of all the old, but simplistic equation, that if every Chinese person were given a refrigerator, the impact on the environment would be disastrous. However, it is equally difficult to imagine the world remaining stable for long if the system prevailed by which some countries were compelled to remain poor in order to protect the world from the impact of unsustainable growth. Consideration of such problems by socially conscious people in the first world is often associated with the adoption of what are perceived as more environmentally friendly lifestyles and an ethical commitment to reducing consumption to far below what one's actual wealth might sustain.

But it has long been realised that levels of individual consumption in the first world rise and fall, even to the extent of causing changes in the economic cycles, without any associated or predictable change in third-world economic well-being. When considering levels of production, many people seem to believe that there is a fixed supply of goods for the world's people, rendering direct the connection between one person's overconsumption and another's deprivation. But the relationship, of course, is much more complex than that.

For one thing, individual actions – especially along different lines or with different emphases – in some senses resemble quantum mechanics in that the slight variations are masked by the direction of the system as a whole. Even conscientious green consumerism is disappointing in its impact if practised by individuals outside a wider and more co-ordinated political context. For a person from the first world to engage in the enterprise of green consumerism in an attempt to reduce negative effects on the environment takes no account of how retailing works. If environmentally friendly goods are not widely and easily available on the market, why would people go out of their way to purchase – at some inconvenience and at a higher price – a product which they could have obtained more easily and more cheaply if they had not been aware of the environmental argument (or chose to ignore it)?

Our 'democratic' freedom under Western capitalism does allow us to act as individuals, even to the extent of making it possible and legal for individuals to shop in an environmentally friendly fashion. But for this to be organised and directed so as to actually have a noticeable and planned impact would require such mass mobilisation and counter-cultural propaganda that it would probably have to be subversive in order to keep the democratic forces from effectively defending themselves against it. Without that, almost any realistic increase, say, in car usage in the third world would make less of a negative environmental impact than would even a small percentage reduction imposed politically and through legislation in the Western countries, in terms of a positive environmental impact.

In fact, the example of the internal combustion engine points to a crucial general consideration. This is that environmental destruction is caused less by actual consumption than by how specific consumables are produced. As Lisa Macdonald (1998) points out, 20 kilometres is the same in Sydney or in Punjab, but the difference is great indeed if the Punjabi travels it by bicycle while the Australian does it by car. Obviously, wealth and consumption are not the same thing. The sort of improvement that urgently needs to be brought about involves a different view of what wealth is. If wealth were widely conceived as being understood in terms of an individual feeling enhanced through the exercise of the social good, it would be possible for wealth to be far more general than it can be at present.

There is no question that we are not merely discussing a 'feel-good' factor here, but are concerned with materially raising the eating and living standards of great masses of poor people to a level consistent with operational definitions of community health. We can do this simply because even present-day technology can already deliver the products to make it possible. Altering the way in which these are distributed would make virtually no further negative environmental impact. Indeed, by eliminating the need for wasteful practices such as widespread deforestation, overfishing, soil degradation and the like, the sum environmental impact would doubtless be positive over time.

This is where the political theories need to come in. In 1976, a seminal book was written by Barry Commoner (*The Poverty of the Planet*), basing much of his analysis on a critique of US capitalism. From 1945 to 1970, US per capita consumption rose 6% while per capita pollution rose by 700% or more! Suppose that US consumption standards could be achieved for the great majority in the third world, but at only a fraction of the environmental cost that it had entailed in the USA. That would certainly be possible, but it would be resisted by people and governments that were tied into the classical market-forces model.

Thus we are faced with a more basic task – altering people's mindset on a very broad scale. But, again, we really do not have any realistic option. Looking at it optimistically, that is the path we will follow – because there is no other – and the broad realisation of this by the world's people will bring it about without protracted revolutionary conflict. A more pessimistic view would see it coming about, but only through direct revolutionary confrontation and protracted upheaval – which itself might well be environmentally disastrous. But the most pessimistic view of all would be that these changes will not come about and the planet will gradually become a write-off, along with all of its inhabitants.

The optimistic view as a solution

How can the profit motive be replaced by a concept of wealth that is measured in terms of satisfaction of actual human needs? Surely, large business corporations will use their power over governments to legitimise the continued production of destructive products. A fixation on short-term profit-making strategies would leave out any consideration of sustainability. What such a consideration implies is that environmentally sustainable methods really are inimical to capitalism.

Many otherwise educated people, especially in the first world, have been conditioned to think that such a proposition is psychologically impossible. References are frequently made to 'human nature', as though that were a constant rather than a variable. But, of course, had such been the case, we would never have evolved as we have. Then again, reference is often made to the 'market place' – a figurative concept that supposedly determines what our social and political arrangements must be to meet 'needs' dictated by 'people's will'. In this, there is much putting of carts before horses, but the argument is obviously compelling, nevertheless.

Let us take transport, for instance. Various convincing arguments based on environmental considerations, reduction in traffic congestion and the like, have been put forward in favour of increased government expenditure on public transport and a proportional withdrawal of its expenditures in facilitating private transport. Arguments against it are based on the sense of 'control' one has over one's movement in the private car as opposed to having to structure one's activities around public transport timetables. But in any big city today, the increasing frequency of huge grid-locked traffic jams and the sheer tension engendered by driving defensively for, say, an hour before starting one's real work each day, is seriously eroding the appeal of the 'control' argument. By and large there is very little empirical reason for believing that people really care about how it is done, but whether they get from A to B comfortably, reliably and on time. Public transport, if it is even handled only moderately well, removes serious stresses from the lives of city dwellers. There is no worry that the car might be vandalised while one is at work. And, indeed, the element of personal control does not have to be lost. In Germany, for instance, car ownership is more widespread than it is in the UK, but use of private cars in urban areas and during the weekdays is far less. Basically, Germans prefer to use public transport in town and private transport for weekend jaunts.

However, the issue cannot be addressed purely at the individual level. Considerable political leadership is required to render public transport a realistic alternative before, say, Londoners will become like Berliners in sufficient numbers to make a difference. At present a test of preferences is not realistic because public transport systems in much of the first world are deliberately run in such a way as to make them non-competitive with private vehicles. The oil industry, to name just one, is able to exert immense pressure on local and national governments to organise their transport spending in such a way as to enhance the private sector.

In his book Commoner (1976) quotes from a 1974 report to a US Senate subcommittee which detailed the planned destruction of electronically powered rail transport in 45 US cities. The principal actors in this assault on public transport were three: General Motors, Standard Oil and the Firestone Tire Company. General Motors bought up the targeted railway companies, dismantled the tracks, substituted General Motors' buses, and then sold the companies to private buyers. People's choices did not get a look in. Similar attacks on the public sector are now commonplace in Eastern Europe, where former communist regimes are being initiated into market forces (Athanasiou, 1996). Any workable social solutions which we eventually evolve to avoid the calamity facing us will probably involve a combination of 'red' and 'green' thinking. By 'red', of course, I refer to some kind of globally feasible socialist economy and by 'green' to communal action consistent with environmental sustainability.

Pre-political Greening

The foregoing may easily strike the reader as a counsel of despair, but that is because we have focused on the link between the well nigh universal urge to be recognised as working for a social good that transcends consumerism and the role of constitutional democratic government. Together with attempts to revamp our social responses, we can consider various organised, but 'pre-political', green initiatives. In the UK, to begin with a negative critique of 'Uncle Tony' and the operational Toryism of the Labour Party, is to impose a crippling sense of defeatism. (Tony Blair, Leader of the British Labour Party, renamed 'New Labour', returned to office in the national elections of 2005.) But, as the German Greens have shown, we must avoid seeing electoral politics as the first objective.

In fact, the German Greens discovered, to their cost and ours, that the green agenda, which matured during the 1960s in bedrooms, cafes and factory canteens, lost its vibrancy and much of its advocacy potential once it became respectable enough to enter government as a party. The road to victory often lies outside parliament. Consider the temporary victories gained by Greenpeace against Shell or the victories of grassroots movements against the Multinational Agreement on Investment. The international power of corporate capital is probably subject to more opposition or actions outside parliament than within it.

Ultimately, of course, particular democratic governments will be forced to accept responsibility by a better-educated and informed public for their lack of response to electoral prompting. It is their acquiescence, if not direct corruption, that has opened up the world's resources (primarily the third world's resources) to exploitation by their own trans-nationals. In this there is considerable scope for optimism, because the knowledge that their supposed representatives in parliament are succumbing to corporate pressures will increasingly lead the people to seek out other sources of power to challenge that. This should provide an opportunity and the time for Greens and Reds alike to establish a presence in the popular mind, a chance for a more hopeful alternative. It is a truism that any party attempting to gain power on a platform of environmental responsibility and of social equity will need to have established dependable roots in the social consciousness.

Can Green political power survive bureaucracy?

It has been said that Reds tend to be so preoccupied with organisation and reliable chains of commands, that their very ideological purity drives them into tightly controlled little splinter groups. If anything, the Greens face the opposite problem. They recognise the importance of grassroots inspiration, but seem to have trouble organising it into a hierarchical structure without killing the spirit of the enterprise. As one well-known Dutch Green explained to me, 'Our philosophical agenda requires us to aim at both social equity and environmental sustainability simultaneously. But at the individual level we can only take on the environment!'

However, this really is a false dichotomy if reduced to operational terms. The two goals are philosophically symbiotic – you cannot have one without the other. This is because the most environmentally friendly way of providing for human need is for everyone to have equal access to what is produced. With respect to access to health, this has been well established by Wilkinson (1996). Over two decades he made a longitudinal study of what variations in people's health occurred when incomes have moved towards equality: the incidence of disease has dropped, while life expectancy has risen. Moreover, by multivariate analysis, he was able to show that these changes were independent of economic growth, better healthcare or even the movement of individual people out of absolute poverty. As Wilkinson (1996) rather starkly put it, 'There are too few people in absolute poverty in any of the first world nations for their death rates to have a significant influence on the statistics!'

Wilkinson points out that since the early 1970s, Japan has moved up from about the 60th percentile with respect to both life expectancy and income distribution to the top in both. Now Japan boasts the highest recorded life expectancy (83 years for women, 80 for men) and also the most egalitarian income distribution in the world. Conversely, while British income distribution worsened drastically throughout the 1980s, producing the most glaring inequalities since 1885, British life expectancy figures also dropped. Since 1985, mortality rates for both sexes and between the ages of 16 and 45 years have risen steadily. Again, multivariate analysis allowed Wilkinson to remove AIDS deaths as a variable and yet the relationship still persisted.

What this means is that in the UK people are dying at an earlier age than they need, not because they do not have enough to survive on, but because the distribution of resources is inequitable. How this can be is a more difficult question to answer. If one has enough money to buy sufficient food, fuel and shelter to stay alive when there is not much variation in incomes, why should this prove harder if many others suddenly become wealthier? Wilkinson argues that it is a matter of social psychology. This would suggest the validity of my comment earlier in this chapter, that people cannot function optimally as individuals. They need approval, and the feeling that they are valued, to relate effectively to the larger community. Being on low income levels obviously devalues a person, decreases their sense of social meaning (and hence their meaning as a person) and can lead to a collapse of self-esteem. It is well-known, of course, that this has a deleterious effect on health. That is a real clinical fact – not a supposition. Such people die of clinically diagnosed pathologies, but a psychologically depressed state renders anyone less able to resist such illnesses.

On this basis, Wilkinson argues that once an adequate level of national productivity has been attained, the most effective way of enhancing public health is not necessarily to produce more, but to aim for equalisation of incomes. In his words: 'This might be expected to improve the quality of life for everyone by improving the social fabric and simultaneously slowing the pace of environmental degradation.'

Such findings lead to strong empirical support to the primary thesis of this chapter that, not only is there a feasible basis for Reds and Greens to pool their objectives, but convincing evidence that they cannot act effectively in isolation from one another. Social justice, equity and respect for the integrity of the environment is the only policy by which global health promotion can become a reality. It is practical, not visionary, and probably our only viable choice.

References

Athanasiou T (1996) *Divided Planet*. Little, Brown & Co, New York, NY.

Brown P (2004) Hydrogen seen as car fuel of the future. *The Guardian*. 10 September.

Chandler D (2004) In just 50 years we could cure our addiction to oil. *New Scientist*. 19 October.

Commoner B (1976) *The Poverty of the Planet*. Alfred Knopf, New York, NY.

Macdonald L (1998) Malign design. *New Internationalist Magazine*. 307: 122–31.

MacDonald T (1984) *Making a New People: education in revolutionary Cuba*. New Star Books, Vancouver, CA.

MacDonald T (1998) *Schooling the Revolution*. Praxis Press, London.

MacDonald T (2000) *Developments in Cuban Healthcare Since 1959*. The Edwin Mellen Press, New York.

MacDonald T (2005) *Third World Health: hostage to first world wealth*. Radcliffe Publishing, Oxford.

Monbiot G (2004) Fuel for nought. *The Guardian*. 23 November. p. 21.

O'Keefe E and Scott-Samuel A (2002) Human rights and wrongs: could health impact assessment help? *Journal of Law, Medicine and Ethics*. 30: 734–8.

Pacala S and Socolow R (2004) 15 ways to reduce oil consumption. *Science*. 305: 698.

Radford T (2005) Biomass fuel 'needs help'. *Guardian*. 8 August.

Ramose M (1999) *African Philosophy Through Ubuntu*. Mond Books, Harare.

Smith L (2005) People's Health Assembly 2. Monthly spotlight. August 2005. *Social Medicine Portal* (Available at www.socialmedicine.org; accessed 4 February 2006.)

Toke D (2004) Alternative Energy Review. Oxford Union debate, 29 November.

Wilkinson R (1996) *Unhealthy Societies: the affliction of inequality*. Routledge, London.

United Nations (2005) *Report on the World Social Situation*. Department of Economic and Social Affairs, Division of Social Policy and Development, New York, NY. www.un.org/esa/socdev/rss/rss.htm. Accessed 15 July 2005.

Usborne D (2005) The US vs. the UN. *The Independent*. 26 August.

Index

Page numbers in *italic* refer to tables

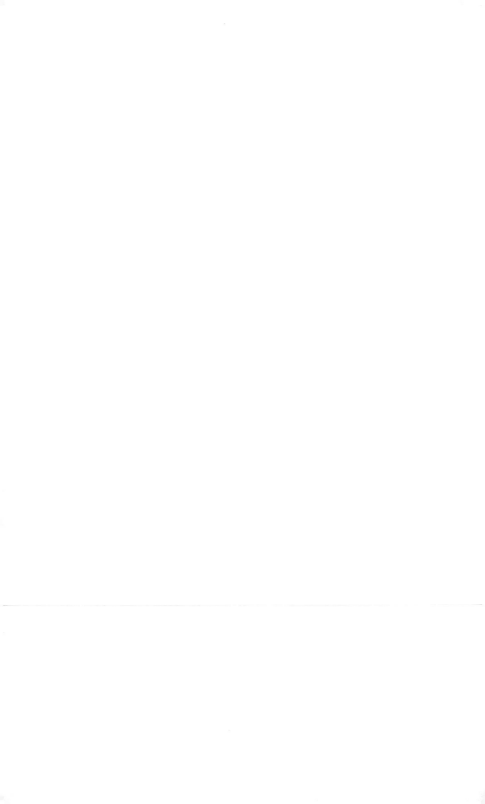